What Is Obsessive Compulsive Disorder

Symptoms of OCD

OCD Test, Treatment for Obsessive Compulsive Disorder, OCD Medication, OCD Symptoms in Children and Adults

Table of contents

Having OCD is like having a bully in my brain...
-Anonymous

ISBN : 978-0-9923922-9-1

Printed by Lightning Source, Victoria

Disclaimer
Although the author and publisher have made every effort to ensure that the information in this book was correct at press time, the author and publisher do not assume and hereby disclaim any liability to any party for any loss, injury, damage or disruption caused by errors or omissions, whether such errors or omissions result from negligence, accident, non-functional websites, or any other cause. Any advice or strategy contained herein may not be suitable for every individual.

Acknowledgements

I would like to extend my sincerest thanks to my friends and family who supported me throughout this journey. I'd like to thank my wife especially for her patience with me throughout my research and writing.

Introduction

In light of the increasing amount of people who receive a diagnosis of OCD, there is definitely a need for more resources on the subject. OCD is often misdiagnosed, causing thousands of people to suffer in silence. The increase in the number of OCD cases is likely due to the fact that healthcare professionals are increasingly aware of this disorder and its consequences on the lives of those affected by it.

While the Internet can be a good source of information, it often presents contradicting or confusing information from more or less reliable sources. Almost any possible claim has been made over the Internet, from miracle drugs to crazy futuristic science. You often need to search dozens of websites in order to find the information you're looking for. When you need to find real information, all condensed up into a neat little package, a book is often the better choice.

The aim of this book is to provide comprehensive information on OCD, including the symptoms and treatments. It provides a list of symptoms in adults, children and toddlers, along with a short self-test to help you identify any OCD symptoms you may have. A general overview of treatments in the last chapter will provide you with insight on the different options that you may be faced with on your journey to conquering OCD.

Living with OCD can be hard, and it often causes significant anxiety and distress. However, it is very treatable. Cognitive behavior therapy (CBT) provides patients with powerful tools to conquer their obsessions and compulsions. This book will explain how CBT works and why it is often the better choice for the treatment of OCD. You will also be taken through a quick summary of medications that your doctor might want to prescribe. A short overview of drug-free treatment options along with some strategies to cope with your OCD completes the chapter.

When it comes to your health, the more you know, the better. Knowing what to expect when you go in for a consultation with a mental health professional or knowing that your OCD can in fact be hidden by depressive symptoms will allow you to better understand the diagnosis and treatment process. If you live with OCD, you likely experience anxiety on a regular basis. Not knowing what to expect could increase your anxiety and hold you back from seeking professional help. In turn, this denies you the precious possibility of receiving treatment that could change your life.

This book is for anyone who thinks they may suffer from OCD, or anyone who is seeking additional information on their symptoms. It was also written for those with loved ones who suffer from OCD or anxiety symptoms. Mental conditions can be difficult to understand for those who have not experienced them firsthand, and being able to shed a little light on the things that are going on in your loved ones' heads can make it easier to accept this illness for what it is: an anxiety disorder that robs you of your life while you try to protect everyone else.

Chapter 1

I do not have OCD OCD OCD.
–Emily Autumn

What is OCD?

Obsessive compulsive disorder (OCD) is a medical disorder which causes you to experience frequent and unwelcome obsessional thoughts which in turn trigger different compulsions or urges. These thoughts cause severe anxiety that can only be relieved by engaging in a ritual or compulsive behavior.

Obsessions usually come in the form of intrusive thoughts about anything from the fear of microbes to the fear of an accident happening to a loved one. Some obsessions can be erotic in nature, with the person becoming overly attached to someone of the same or opposite sex. This goes way beyond love; the obsession can fuel extreme jealousy and suicidal thoughts.

Compulsions are performed over and over again in a ritualistic or repetitive manner. These behaviors actually have a purpose: they temporarily relieve the obsessive thoughts. For example, if you have an uncanny fear of being robbed, you will check that all the windows and doors are locked a dozen times before leaving the house. This temporarily relieves the obsessive thoughts that constantly occur about someone who could possibly walk in through an unlocked door and steal from the house. Someone with an irrational fear of contamination could spend most of their waking time scrubbing and disinfecting the house to try to get rid of every last germ.

Engaging in a compulsive behavior temporarily relieves anxiety, but at the same time it reinforces the obsession. For example, if you're absolutely convinced that your teeth will rot and fall out if you don't brush them enough, you may

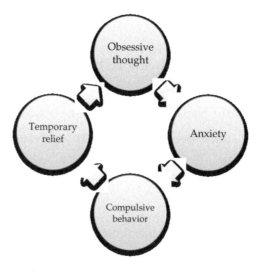

The obsession-compulsion cycle

start engaging in excessive tooth brushing. In turn, this behavior will damage enamel and push back gums, causing root cavities and other problems. Your obsessive thoughts about tooth brushing will come back even stronger because those cavities, in your mind, are caused by insufficient brushing. This creates a vicious circle of obsession and compulsion.

Most OCD symptoms fall into four main categories. Each category contains hundreds of different types of symptoms. Bad things happening to you or your loved ones is usually a strong recurrent theme in obsessive thoughts. For this reason, compulsions are often focused on preventing potential negative events, whether it is contamination, accidents or disease.

- **Checking** involves excessive verification of anything from locked doors to alarm clock settings. People feel compelled to check something an unreasonable amount of times in order to prevent a potential catastrophe. Sometimes, compulsive checking behaviors involve calling or texting loved ones multiple times a day to make sure they are okay.

- The fear of **contamination** prompts behaviors from the second type of OCD. These behaviors include excessive cleaning, disinfecting, hand washing, bathing and anything that can possibly help prevent the spreading of germs. Someone with a fear of germs is often unable to use public restrooms, touch door handles in public places or eat outside of their home.

- **Hoarding** objects in an excessive manner is also typical of OCD. Between 18 and 42 percent of people who suffer from OCD have hoarding behaviors. Severe hoarding can prevent normal activities because the bed, the shower, the kitchen table and other living areas are filled with piles of clothes, newspaper or other objects. This often stems from the fear of making the wrong decision about whether to keep or toss a certain object.

- **Ruminations and intrusive thoughts** are slightly different because they often don't involve physical symptoms such as rituals. Ruminations are obsessive and lengthy contemplation of different religious, metaphysical or philosophical themes. For example, a person could spend unreasonable amounts of time thinking about life after death or the nature of the universe.

  Intrusive thoughts are involuntary recurring thoughts about a particular theme. For example, some people have obsessive doubts about a partner's faithfulness and constantly search for proof of cheating. Certain intrusive thoughts are superstitious in nature. For instance, some people have to do everything in multiples of three, while others avoid everything yellow because they think it is bad luck. A common theme for intrusive thoughts is the fear of not being a good person or not being devout enough.

Who is affected by OCD?

In any given year, approximately 2.2 million American adults struggle with obsessive compulsive disorder. This represents one percent of the population. OCD affects half as many children and teenagers. This means that an average elementary or middle school contains four to five children who suffer from OCD. In a large high school, as many as 20 young people can face the challenges of OCD on a daily basis.

The median age of onset is 19 years old, but it begins much earlier in a large proportion of people. In fact, most adults who live with OCD have had symptoms since they were children. Although obsessive compulsive disorder affects men and women equally, boys are more likely to develop it before puberty. Onset after 35 years of age is very rare.

Physiological and psychological causes of OCD

There is currently no known cause for OCD. However, there are several theories that point to a variety of factors involved in its development. OCD is most likely a mixture of several physical, environmental and psychological factors.

Genetics

Having a family member who suffers from a type of OCD seems to increase the likelihood of developing the disorder. For example, up to 30% of teenagers with OCD had at least one member of their immediate family who was prone to obsessive symptoms. Obsessive symptoms can include various disorders on the OCD spectrum: body dysmorphic disorder, which is excessive worrying over small or imagined physical defects; hypochondria, an excessive fear of having a serious illness despite professional reassurance; binge eating or anorexia; and trichotillamonia, a compulsive behavior which causes the person to pull out their own or other people's hair.

OCD does not appear to be purely genetic because identical twins will not necessarily both develop the disorder. If one parent has OCD, there seems to be a 2% to 8% chance that each child will also have it. This could be partly due to genetics and partly to household environment such as eating habits.

Physical causes

Brain scans done on people with OCD show that they often have malfunctions that affects communication between different parts of the brain, prompting inappropriate responses when anxiety arises. These parts of the brain affected by structural abnormalities do not belong to the "logical" brain and cannot be reasoned with. This explains why OCD sufferers are often aware of everything but feel like they cannot control it.

Normally, the brain is wired to send and receive signals that prompt us to react to certain impulses. For example, after you have used the washroom, your brain sends a signal that it's time to wash your hands in order to remove potentially harmful germs. It creates an impulse, to which you respond by walking over to the sink and turning on the faucet. This is all done without the need to really think about it. This particular brain circuit stops being stimulated after you have accomplished the action, ending the feedback loop and letting you to go back to your activities.

In people with OCD, this feedback loop is broken and the brain can no longer turn off or ignore impulses from this particular circuit. The impulse therefore remains even after completing the action, causing them to repeat the same action over and over again. They are aware that they just finished washing their hands, but they cannot explain nor control the resulting impulsion to continue.

Recently, OCD has been linked to low levels of serotonin, a chemical inside the brain which is responsible for carrying information from one neuron to another. When serotonin levels are too low, the brain reacts differently to anxiety. Normally, unnecessary thoughts are naturally filtered out but because of low levels of serotonin, they are interpreted as "danger signals" and cause high levels of anxiety. Low serotonin also causes depressive thoughts such as guilt and excessive worry, which all comes together with high anxiety to create some seriously disturbing thought loops.

Infection

Some "strep throat" infections have been known to cause sudden and severe OCD in some people. However, this happens very rarely and seems to affect people who had a genetic predisposition. In other words, it's more like a trigger than an actual cause. In these cases, OCD is probably the result of the body accidentally attacking healthy cells while trying to combat the infection, resulting in tissue damage inside the brain. If this damage occurs in the areas associated with OCD, symptoms can develop within a few weeks.

Guilt

Some children learn to feel guilty and responsible from a very young age. These feelings are strongly involved in many OCD cases. If a child constantly feels like a bad person for having certain thoughts or doing certain things, he might become obsessed with becoming perfect, preventing accidents or trying to repress "bad" thoughts.

Facts on OCD

OCD symptoms can change over time. Sometimes, a child will engage in a certain compulsive behavior and later on, he or she might develop a new compulsion. These obsessions and compulsions can come and go or they can be constant.

Until recently, OCD was thought to be a pretty rare disorder. This is due to the fact that people who live with OCD often become masters at hiding their symptoms from others to avoid being perceived as crazy. They will perform their rituals in private and avoid situations that are likely to trigger them in public. Sometimes, they will integrate their compulsions with their daily activities in order to draw less attention to them. This secrecy surrounding OCD symptoms has kept the disorder hidden from both family members and health professionals for years.

OCD behaviors can be logically tied to the fear they represent. Someone who is afraid of accidentally sending inappropriate emails might read everything dozens of time before sending it to make sure it won't offend the recipient. Other times, the behaviors have absolutely no connection to the fear, like the true story of a young man who was unable to move from his chair before midnight on the off chance that someone might get hurt if he did. He knew it made no sense but in his mind, it *could* happen and he didn't want to take the chance.

Today, health professionals as well as the general public have greater awareness of this disorder. Treatment options are also more promising, encouraging affected people to seek treatment. Although the general perception of OCD has greatly improved, it is still clouded by stereotypes and false assumptions. Many people think of OCD as excessive hand washing, but there are hundreds of different types of obsessions and compulsions.

How was OCD discovered?

OCD has probably existed for a while, but strange behavior was not attributed to medical disorders until very recently. In the 17th century, some writings referred to OCD in the form of people who spoke inappropriate things in church or who struggled with naughty and blasphemous thoughts made worse by their attempts at suppressing them.

Two centuries later, the modern concept of OCD started to evolve as distinction was made between delusions, obsession, compulsions and neurosis. The disorder went through a variety of names, and dozens of theories emerged on its causes. It was finally regarded as a mental disorder rather than an affliction caused by a lack of religious faith. Still, people with OCD and other mental disorders were often considered crazy.

In the 20th century, it became known as "obsessive compulsive disorder" and the concept was more clearly defined. We can't say that anyone discovered OCD; it is the result of several centuries of studying human behavior. Recent technology now allows us to have a look inside the brain of those who suffer from mental disorders, potentially allowing us to find some biological clues that would spark the development of new medications and treatments.

OCD and other mental disorders

One very common recurrent though in people with OCD is the fear of schizophrenia. Random words get stuck in their head, strange thoughts pop in their mind and they engage in internal dialogue. The obsessive component of OCD will cause them to spend too much time thinking about these things. OCD can cause paranoia, delusions and phobias and create a thought loop that makes the person afraid of becoming psychotic or losing their mind. However, these are all normal manifestations of OCD.

Sometimes, OCD comes with another mental disorder such as depression, anxiety and bipolar disorder. In people who live with these dual disorders, the obsessive compulsive disorder often goes unnoticed and thus, untreated.

Depression and OCD often go hand in hand; this is particularly challenging to deal with as depression affects motivation and self-esteem. As many as three out of four people with OCD suffer from co-occurring depression. Usually, depression will have to be taken care of before starting an OCD recovery program since this type of therapy is often very emotionally involving.

What it's like to live with OCD

> *Getting dressed in the morning was tough, because I had a routine, and if I didn't follow the routine, I'd get anxious and would have to get dressed again. I always worried that if I didn't do something, my parents were going to die. I'd have these terrible thoughts of harming my parents. I knew that was completely irrational, but the thoughts triggered more anxiety and more senseless behavior. Because of the time I spent on rituals, I was unable to do a lot of things that were important to me.*
> —Anonymous

People who live with OCD usually overestimate their role in disease and accident prevention. This causes tremendous stress, anxiety and guilt. As with many anxiety disorders, the perceived threat of an obsessive thought is much higher than its realistic probability or consequences. For example, the fear of accidentally burning down your house could lead you to check the light switches and appliances fifty times before going to work. In your mind, this will prevent any possible fires from happening. However, the realistic chances of a fire actually happening are very slim. Still, you might feel guilty and anxious if you don't carry out this ritual every time.

Friends or relatives of people with OCD often feel overwhelmed by their ritualistic behaviors. A husband whose wife compulsively checks the taps before leaving the house because she's afraid of causing a flood can feel impatient and frustrated. A mother who calls her son five times a day to make sure he's still alive and healthy can make him feel suffocated and drive him away. This will reinforce the mother's thoughts that she needs to take better care of her son and feed her OCD.

For this reason, those who live with OCD can have difficulty maintaining healthy relationships. It is often hard for people around them to accept their irrational behaviors and even harder to bring them up. The person with OCD already feels guilty and anxious about something, and being told that their behavior is irritating to others can cause massive distress. At the same time, the excessive behaviors drive others away, fueling more potential catastrophic scenarios of accidents, rejection and death.

Keeping a job when you live with OCD can often be very challenging. In severe cases, the compulsive rituals can last for hours and cause you to be late for work. If the fear of germs takes over at the office, you can spend hours washing your hands and become very unproductive. Most employers do not tolerate this type of behavior because the lost productivity is bad for business.

Most people with obsessive compulsive disorder are consciously aware that their behaviors are irrational. Often, they'll try to stop but their anxiety takes over. Their logical mind tells them that spending so much time sanitizing the house is a little excessive, but they are incapable of stopping because they profoundly want to prevent their loved ones from getting sick.

Doubt and uncertainty feed OCD, and those emotions often cause irrational behaviors that defy even the strongest willpower. Basically, having OCD can be compared to having low tolerance to uncertainty. Since uncertainty is a normal part of life, these people go through significant stress on a daily basis. Many people who live with OCD are ridden with guilt when something bad happens because they were unable to prevent it.

On top of the stress brought on by their condition, OCD sufferers have to live with a debilitating disorder that significantly interferes with their daily life. Their quality of life is often reduced as they are plagued with anxious thoughts and spend most of their waking day trying to prevent catastrophes. The shame experienced by people who don't fully understand the nature of their compulsions can stop them from enjoying normal things such as dating, intimacy and social activities.

When OCD takes the form of recurrent intrusive thoughts of murder, cannibalism, racism, animal abuse and other horrific things, it can deeply affect self-perception. Not only can those thoughts be awful on their own, but the person stuck with these persistent thoughts often feels like a really bad person for even having them. The inability to share these thoughts with people around them makes them feel alone and crazy.

As far as the social perception of OCD goes, it has definitely changed over the years. While it is getting better in terms of social acceptance, it often gets ridiculed, especially with the modern Internet culture. Several "memes" targeted at people with OCD circulate on the Web and they can be quite offensive to those who actually live with the condition. People share quotes and stereotypes through social media, and sometimes OCD is shrugged off as kids who like to eat their M&Ms in a specific color order or someone who needs to set the television volume in multiples of five. The truth is, it's far more than that.

OCD in the media

The media has a special way of portraying just about every mental disorder in a very clichéd manner. Unfortunately, OCD does not escape this fact. On TV, people with OCD are always checking, cleaning, rearranging or whatever compulsion the producers decided to bestow upon them. Rarely do we see anything about the agony experienced by these people with recurrent thoughts of very horrible things.

We don't get to see their troubling thought loop about accidentally killing their entire family because their books were not arranged in perfect order. We don't really see any TV characters who avoid public places because they are afraid of becoming sexually aroused in the presence of children. They don't show us how simply thinking about that possibility can make these characters feel extremely guilty. It is difficult to portray these kinds of things on TV, and some thoughts could even be too disturbing to many viewers. This perpetuates the myth that OCD is excessive hand washing and minor annoying or funny quirks.

Medical brochures and textbooks describe OCD very factually as a disorder involving obsessions and compulsions. For example, "recurrent and intrusive thoughts" can mean just about anything and certainly does not conjure images of horrific things. While this description of symptoms is true, it hardly does justice to what really goes on in these people's heads. For these reasons, OCD is still widely misunderstood and often goes unrecognized.

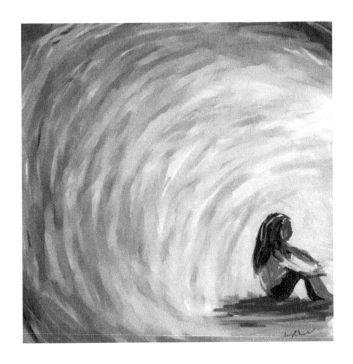

One thing which I can't stress enough is that OCD is completely nonsensical and will not listen to reason. This is one of the most frightening things about having it. I knew that to anyone I told, there are Salvador Dali paintings that make more sense.

—Joe Wells, *Touch and Go Joe: An Adolescent's Experience of OCD*

Chapter 2

I swear, I am like, soooo OCD....

Recognizing OCD symptoms

OCD symptoms can be divided into two main categories: obsessive thoughts and compulsive behaviors. Symptoms from both categories are usually present, although a small percentage of people don't openly manifest any compulsive behaviors. However, compulsions are a response to obsessive thoughts and they are necessary to feed the OCD cycle. For these rare people, rituals take the shape of thoughts and mental compulsions.

When they are bombarded by obsessive thoughts, usually of sexual, religious or violent nature, they respond with a compulsion that takes place in their head. For instance, a woman who's obsessed with not being a good enough person could spend much of her time silently apologizing to God. She could bargain with herself, seek constant reassurance from those around her, give money to charity or any other behavior that can convince her of her pious and kind nature. The time she spends talking to God in her head and promising herself to give up sweets in exchange for forgiveness are not very noticeable. From the outside, it could appear as though she has no compulsions. These silent compulsions are known as "covert compulsions".

Obsessive and intrusive thoughts
- Fear of contamination (getting contaminated or contaminating others)
- Fear of causing harm to yourself, loved ones or strangers
- Unwanted graphic thoughts and images of violent or sexual nature
- Excessive worrying about religion or morality
- Fear of losing things or not having something that you need
- Order and symmetry, where everything has to line up, be symmetrical or in a certain order
- Superstition, where there is excessive focus on some things that are considered lucky or unlucky
- Doubt, where you constantly think you've done something wrong or made a mistake

Compulsive behaviors
- Excessive checking of appliances, locks, windows, brakes, alarm clocks and other things
- Compulsive texting and calling of loved ones to make sure they are safe

- Doing everything in multiples of a certain number, two and three being very common
- Compulsive counting, tapping or any other behavior aimed at reducing anxiety
- Excessive washing and cleaning
- Extreme orderliness, like sorting things in alphabetical order or facing all the hangers in your closet in a certain direction
- Severe hoarding of objects, to the point of disrupting daily life
- Excessive praying or mental rituals
- Constant need of reassurance, such as confessing all your horrible intrusive thoughts in order to be told that you would never do such a thing

Obsessive belief	Compulsion
☐ Fear of contamination (germs, being dirty)	☐ Compulsive hand washing and showering
☐ Symmetry, order, exactness	☐ Doing things in multiples of two or three, repeating rituals
☐ Fear of terrible things happening (fire, burglary, flood)	☐ Checking appliances, light switches, doors, locks

An obsessive belief triggers a compulsion

Here are some examples of unwanted obsessive thoughts that could severely disturb a person with OCD. Obviously there are thousands of different possibilities, but the common characteristic about these obsessive thoughts is that they cause high levels of anxiety. This anxiety can only be relieved temporarily by engaging in certain rituals which may or may not be related to the obsession.

- Sexual thoughts about a religious figure
- Thoughts about stabbing someone, drowning a baby or kicking an animal
- Thoughts that if a certain thing is not done, people will die or get hurt
- Thoughts about being bisexual or homosexual
- Fear of running over someone with a car without realizing it
- Inappropriate thoughts about having sex with family members
- Fear of having a serious physical or mental illness

We can certainly see why these intrusive thoughts would cause fear and distress in people who experience them on a regular basis. However, if you are having these violent, inappropriate or otherwise disturbing thoughts, it does not make you a bad person. It does not make you crazy, insane, dangerous or evil. These thoughts are symptoms of a mental disorder that affects over one percent of people. They are very difficult to live with, and you could be scared of losing control and acting on these impulsions. This is very normal and it can be treated.

What OCD isn't

It is important to remember that everyone can exhibit a certain amount of obsessive or compulsive traits. This does not mean that we all have OCD. Enjoying a clean, orderly house is not on the same level as scrubbing the walls twice a day. Being in complete love with a movie actor and having his picture all over your room, or being uncomfortable wearing jewelry that doesn't match your outfit are not signs of OCD.

OCD is NOT:

- Collecting coins, stamps, stones, sports memorabilia
- Compulsive shopping and gambling
- Compulsive drinking, eating and lying
- Obsessions with having sex, masturbating, working out or other pleasurable activities
- Crushing on a celebrity
- Minor quirks such as always eating a certain color of M&Ms last
- Obsessive Compulsive Personality Disorder
- Generalized Anxiety Disorder

Hoarding versus collecting

Some people have impressive collections of stamps, stuffed animals or any other item they enjoy. This does not compare to the hoarding characteristic that often accompanies OCD. Compulsive hoarding happens when a person collects worthless trash and is afraid to discard it because something bad could happen. These scenarios often involve someone getting hurt or falling sick as a result of throwing away the junk. Sometimes, it could also be the fear of getting rid of something that could prove extremely useful in the future. The person's house is filled with these items to the point that sometimes, it is impossible to use the bathtub or the furniture.

Addiction behaviors versus OCD

Compulsive shopping, gambling, lying or eating are completely different from OCD. They belong to a category of disorders known as *impulse control disorders.* You get an impulse ("Oh gee, I really must get some new clothes even if I spent half my paycheck on shoes yesterday"). The impulse could be compared to a craving. It does not stem from anxiety and obsessive thoughts, but purely from seeking a certain emotion. The activity, such as sex, gambling or eating, provides pleasure. It becomes problematic when you have a very hard time resisting the perspective of indulging in your addiction. Obviously, impulse control disorders can lead to distress and a variety of psychological problems.

Minor quirks versus compulsive behaviors

Everyone has a unique personality, and we each have some quirks that distinguish us from others. Color-coding your closet, having a specific face-washing ritual at night, being uncomfortable at the idea of foods touching each other on your plate or always feeding your pets in a certain order is not OCD. Some people have even stranger habits such as always using a specific cup to drink milk and another for juice, eating the peanut butter Reese Puffs before the chocolate ones, or spinning their plate clockwise while only eating the food directly in front of them. These behaviors, while certainly odd and a bit compulsive, are not OCD if they do not stem from obsessions and anxiety.

OCD versus Generalized Anxiety Disorder

Generalized anxiety disorder (GAD) and OCD share many common symptoms. People with GAD are filled with worry and often suffer from insomnia because of their anxious thoughts. GAD can become very severe and stop the person from functioning normally. Although GAD causes exaggerated worry and excessive concerns over things like money, family members' health and difficulties at work, there is no ritual following the thoughts that trigger anxiety.

Another key difference between GAD and OCD is the type of thoughts that cause the person to worry. Those with GAD tend to worry about everything in most aspects of their lives; they anticipate disasters and often panic if they believe they will be unable to handle them. In people with OCD, the worries tend to be confined to one or a few areas of their lives. In other words, their thoughts revolve around their obsession(s) rather than anything that could go wrong in the run of a day. Unlike GAD sufferers, those with OCD engage in their rituals in order to prevent them from panicking when they feel overwhelmed.

OCPD versus OCD

Obsessive compulsive personality disorder can seem very close to OCD, but one is an anxiety disorder and one is a personality disorder. OCPD often has you thinking of your behavior as desirable: you love spending long periods of time cleaning your house in order to keep it immaculate. You spend hours recopying all your notes to make them perfectly tidy because you can't stand when they are messy. People with OCPD often get annoyed if somebody disturbs their orderly and neat space. They are also characteristically preoccupied with cleanliness, control and perfectionism.

The difference with OCD is that OCPD behaviors are not the result of fear and anxiety. They are performed with the goal of being a good, competent, clean and orderly person. If the ritual cannot be accomplished, the person feels upset and annoyed, but certainly not terrorized. They think of their behavior as normal and acceptable.

OCD is...

The driving force of OCD is the fear that something bad will happen, whether it is actually likely or not. This is what triggers the compulsions, which are aimed at protecting yourself or the people around you. Any compulsive behavior without an obsessional trigger is the result of another disorder. Sometimes, these non-OCD compulsions are minor and other times they cause significant distress. The gravity of these behaviors is not what defines OCD.

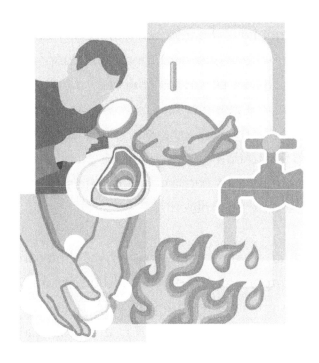

What characterizes OCD is the presence of an obsession-anxiety-compulsion cycle. OCD occupies a large amount of your time and has you constantly scared of the consequences of not carrying out your rituals. You are not *happy* with the obsessive thoughts and the compulsive behaviors certainly don't feel normal. You really want these fears, doubts and thoughts to go away, and you really want to stop doing all those rituals, but you can't. This is real OCD.

OCD symptoms in children

While adults are generally aware of their OCD behavior, children do not have the introspection ability to distinguish between normal behavior and the rituals they feel the need to perform. This often causes children to be embarrassed, thinking they are going crazy. In most cases, they will not tell adults about their bizarre thoughts and behaviors. This can lead to frustration on the children's part when they find themselves unable to perform their rituals because of the rules imposed by their parents.

Because children are usually secretive about their OCD habits, it is important that parents and other adults keep an eye out for signs and symptoms. Often, these signs will be very subtle. The symptoms of OCD in children are similar to those of adults, but because they don't willingly talk about it, the disorder can go unnoticed for a long time.

There are a few observable signs that can help parents get some clues about their child's condition. While these signs do not indicate OCD on their own, they can be a starting point for dialogue.

- Raw, chapped or dry hands from excessive washing
- Unusually high utility bills
- Excessive use of paper towels or soap
- Holes erased through homework or test papers
- Unproductive hours spent doing homework
- Requests for others to repeat certain phrases or answer the same questions in a certain way
- Persistent fear of illness or germs
- Unexplained increase in laundry
- Excessive time spent getting ready for bed or school
- Constant fear that something will happen to a loved one
- Always checking on the health of family members
- Throwing frequent temper tantrums when things cannot be done a certain way
- Sudden drop in test and homework grades

Such unexplained behaviors should be discussed with the child in a delicate manner. When talking to a child about something such as OCD, it is important to be non-judgmental and kind. Being able to talk to an adult who understands and reassures the child can bring great comfort. Sometimes, the adult will have to open up first in order to get the child to talk. Engaging in meaningful dialogue will make the child realize that other people can feel the same way.

It should be noted that children often go through a phase of ritualistic behavior such as a specific bedtime routine, collecting special objects, having a lucky charm or sorting toys in a distinct manner. This behavior is normal and should not be interpreted as OCD. The difference lies in the impact that the behaviors have on the child's life. OCD behaviors will interfere with the child's life at school and/or at home.

For children with OCD, their ritualistic behavior can significantly affect their daily life in many different ways. Their grades can start dropping as a result of constant intrusive thoughts that make them unable to concentrate. Sometimes, they turn in assignments late because they spent an unusual amount of time on it. Their self-esteem can drop significantly as they are bombarded with scary thoughts that make them feel crazy. They can start withdrawing from regular activities. They can throw a tantrum when the anxiety reaches an unbearable level, especially if they cannot engage in their ritual to get some relief.

Children with OCD often feel misunderstood and alone. When engaging in a conversation with them, the focus should be on their feelings. In other words, what drives the behavior. For example, children should not be scolded for using up too much soap or water, as it can decrease the chances of having them confess the thoughts behind it. Instead, a more gentle approach can be used, such as "Mommy noticed that you use a lot of soap to wash your hands often. Are you afraid of something? Are you worried that germs will make you sick?"

In order to investigate a little further into the child's mind, some other questions can be asked:

- What happens if you don't do [ritual]?
- Are there some scary thoughts in your head?
- Do you notice when you do everything in multiples of three?
- Are you worried that bad things will happen to the people you love?
- Do you feel better after doing [ritual]?

Throughout the conversation, the child should be reassured that he is not crazy, and that other people sometimes have the same thoughts. Children often don't grasp the concept of psychiatric treatment and as a result, usually think that their condition cannot be corrected. Telling them that a special doctor can help them make the scary thoughts go away can be enough to give them hope.

OCD symptoms in toddlers

The symptoms of OCD in toddlers can be very hard to detect. OCD often manifests itself as an obsession with organizing things, counting or doing things in a specific order. Sometimes, toddlers will ask a question repeatedly in the hopes of receiving the same answer every time. Once again, toddlers go through phases of organizing things as they learn to distinguish shapes and colors. However, if the behavior is done with the intent of relieving anxiety, it is not part of normal child development. Toddlers can also refuse to go to bed because they are scared of something or worry excessively while in bed.

Toddlers are too young to be diagnosed with OCD. However, if anxiety and OCD-like behaviors interfere with the toddler's life, seeking professional help could still be a good solution. Behavior modification therapy can help take care of the early signs of OCD. The earlier OCD behavior and anxiety are treated, the better the chances of conquering the disease.

The OCD severity spectrum

Just like there is more than one type of OCD, there is more than one way it can affect your daily life. When talking about the severity of OCD, the main criteria is its impact on your activities at home, at work, at school and in social situations.

Mild OCD

The mild form of OCD can be thought of as an *inconvenience*. It is very annoying, but it does not disrupt your activities. You are still able to function at home and at work, and you are still capable of maintaining healthy relationships. You have goals and you are able to pursue them.

Moderate OCD

Moderate OCD is *problematic*. This is when difficulties begin to appear at work or at home. Your OCD occupies much of your time and it affects your performance during your daily activities. Your relationships with others are suffering as a consequence. You find it difficult to have goals and objectives because your OCD takes up much of your time.

Severe OCD

Severe OCD is *debilitating*. You are pretty much unable to function at work and at school, and daily tasks are very difficult to accomplish. You spend most of your time thinking about your obsessions or engaging in your compulsive behaviors. Your significant relationships are affected, and you may already have lost most of your friends. You generally have little interest in pursuing goals and long-term projects.

Mild
- Daily functioning unaltered or slightly affected
- Relationships not affected or slightly affected
- Goals and purposes

Moderate
- Daily functioning significantly altered
- Relationships significantly affected
- Difficulty with goals and purposes

Severe
- Unable to function in daily activities
- Unable to maintain significant relationships
- No interest in goals and purposes

The OCD severity spectrum

Chapter 3

When the disease is known it is half cured.
— Erasmus Colloquies

OCD diagnosis process

Despite the increasing awareness about OCD, physicians often misdiagnose it. This is why knowing your symptoms and taking a screening self-test can help your doctor identify OCD. It takes an average of 14 to 17 years to obtain a diagnosis of obsessive compulsive disorder. If you hide your symptoms from your doctor out of embarrassment, you are denying yourself the opportunity to receive an accurate diagnosis that will allow you to receive an effective treatment for this common medical condition.

First, your doctor will want to rule out any other condition that could cause your symptoms. He will proceed to a physical exam to make sure you are not suffering from complications related to your symptoms. This will also allow him to check for diseases that could cause similar symptoms to what you are experiencing. He may order some lab tests to check for alcohol, drugs, thyroid functions and blood cell count.

Once all the possible physical causes have been ruled out, your doctor will refer you to a mental health specialist. These specialists can be therapists, psychiatrists or psychologists and they are trained in recognizing the symptoms of several mental disorders. Although it may sound scary, a consultation with a mental health specialist is very common and it can greatly help you.

There is a certain social stigma attached to those who see a "shrink". However, there is no need to be ashamed of seeking help for your medical condition. Seeing a psychiatrist or psychologist is like seeing a doctor for your brain. It does not mean you are crazy or dangerous. In fact, many people consult mental health specialists for anxiety, depression, OCD, psychotic symptoms and other conditions. Your therapist will work with you to help you take control of your symptoms and live a normal life.

Your mental health specialist will ask you some questions regarding your symptoms, such as when they appeared, how they manifest themselves and how you deal with them. All the questions they ask you have a purpose, even if they seem unrelated. Everything you tell your therapist is strictly confidential and will not be shared with anyone who's not involved in your specific case. Sometimes, this psychological evaluation will require the specialist to talk to your family or friends, with your permission.

After gathering enough information, your doctor will often be able to establish a diagnostic. Mental health professionals have reference books which guide them in their diagnostic process, making it easier for them to match your symptoms to a certain condition. However, OCD can be confusing to diagnose because it shares many symptoms with depression, schizophrenia, obsessive compulsive personality disorder, generalized anxiety disorder and other mental illnesses.

The more honest you are about what you are going through, the more your therapist can pinpoint the source of your symptoms. It is understandably difficult to admit that you have recurring images of stabbing someone, inappropriate sexual thoughts or illogical thought processes. These mental health professionals are committed to helping you and they will not judge you for telling the truth. In most cases, they have "seen it all" (or almost) and will not be shocked by your disturbing images and impulses.

OCD diagnosis criteria

Unlike physical illnesses, OCD cannot be diagnosed by running a blood test or examining something under the microscope. OCD diagnosis involves a long talk between you and your doctor so that he can get a good idea of what's going on in your head and its impact on your life. He will then compare your symptoms to those in the Diagnostic and Statistical Manual of Mental Disorders (DSM).

To establish a diagnosis of OCD, you must meet the following criteria from the DSM:

- Your symptoms have been going on for at least 2 weeks;
- You must have either obsessions, compulsions or both;
- These obsessions and compulsions are time-consuming (more than 1 hour per day) or interfere significantly with your daily activities;
- The symptoms are not better explained by another disorder such as depression, schizophrenia or drug use;
- You cannot resist at least one obsession or compulsion, even if you manage to have some control over other symptoms.

Obsessions

- Recurrent, persistent and unwelcome thoughts, images or impulses that cause distress and anxiety;

- You try to ignore these thoughts, impulses or images or you try to neutralize them by performing another action (ritual);
- You may or may not realize that these obsessional ideas are not real.

Compulsions
- Repetitive behaviors that you feel driven to perform, or repetitive mental acts such as counting or praying silently;
- These behaviors are performed with the goal of reducing anxiety brought on by intrusive thoughts and images;
- The behaviors do not provide pleasure, or are not done with the goal of pleasure;
- They are acknowledged as excessive or unreasonable, or they are completely unrelated to the problem they are trying to address.

OCD symptoms self-test

This little self-test, inspired from several resources on the Web, can help you find out if you have some OCD symptoms. This tool is not scientific and its purpose is not to establish a diagnosis. You can rank high on this test without having OCD, or you could suffer from OCD with only one or two symptoms that bother you.

Read the following questions and answer "Yes" or "No" to each question. Think about your life in the past month and whether you've experienced the symptom or not. Be honest, as the goal of this exercise is to help you identify OCD symptoms in your everyday behavior. Once you are done, examine your answers. If you have checked "Yes" to several questions and "Yes" to at least one of the questions in the last section (Impact on daily life), you may suffer from OCD. The best way to really know is to consult a specialist.

The last section is particularly important in order to evaluate your symptoms. Everyone can suffer from one or more OCD-like symptoms but as long as it doesn't affect their daily life or as long as they can control it, it is not really a cause for concern. When the intrusive thoughts and compulsive behaviors start affecting your life, such as making you late for work, reducing the amount of time you can spend with your family or causing crippling anxiety, you will most likely wish to seek treatment.

Identifying OCD symptoms and their impact

Intrusive thoughts

In the past MONTH, have you been bothered by any recurring and unwanted thoughts about:

1. Contamination by germs, dirt or chemicals, or mental contamination by ideas, beliefs or opinions?
   - ❑ Yes
   - ❑ No
2. Having a serious disease such as cancer, AIDS or schizophrenia?
   - ❑ Yes
   - ❑ No
3. Needing to arrange or keep things in perfect order?
   - ❑ Yes
   - ❑ No
4. Images of death, accidents, disasters and other horrible events?
   - ❑ Yes
   - ❑ No
5. Inappropriate religious or sexual thoughts?
   - ❑ Yes
   - ❑ No

Excessive worry

In the past MONTH, have you been worrying a lot about the possibility of terrible things happening such as:

6. Fire, burglary, flooding or having a car accident?
   ❑ Yes
   ❑ No

7. Accidentally hurting someone you love or a complete stranger (like running over a pedestrian with your car or saying something hurtful)?
   ❑ Yes
   ❑ No

8. Spreading an illness such as AIDS or mononucleosis?
   ❑ Yes
   ❑ No

9. Losing something important or valuable?
   ❑ Yes
   ❑ No

10. A loved one getting harmed or sick because you didn't do what you had to do?
    ❑ Yes
    ❑ No

Compulsive behavior

In the past MONTH, have you felt irresistible urges to do certain things over and over or in a specific way, such as:

11. Excessive washing, cleaning or grooming?
    ❑ Yes
    ❑ No

12. Excessive verification of windows, doors, locks, lights, faucets, car brakes or other things?

    ❑ Yes

    ❑ No

13. Counting, arranging, putting in order or evening-up objects?

    ❑ Yes

    ❑ No

14. Collecting useless objects because you are afraid of throwing out something that could be useful?

    ❑ Yes

    ❑ No

15. Repeating a certain behavior a set number of times or until it feels right? (getting up from a chair, brushing your teeth, going through a doorway, etc.)

    ❑ Yes

    ❑ No

16. Excessive time spent rereading or rewriting emails, letters, homework and tests?

    ❑ Yes

    ❑ No

17. A compulsive need to touch objects or people?

    ❑ Yes

    ❑ No

18. Needing to confess some of your thoughts or actions, or seeking constant reassurance that you did something correctly?

    ❑ Yes

❑ No

19. Avoiding certain colors, numbers, letters or symbols because they are associated with unpleasant thoughts, memories or events? (For example, avoiding the number 5 because your mother died when you were 5 years old and you feel it was your fault.)

❑ Yes

❑ No

20. Needing to examine your body on a regular basis to make sure you are not sick?

❑ Yes

❑ No

Impact on daily life

21. Do you feel as though you have NO CONTROL over your obsessive thoughts or compulsive behaviors?

❑ Yes

❑ No

22. Do you feel like it takes you much longer than other people to accomplish certain tasks such as taking a shower, locking the door, driving to the store or writing an email?

❑ Yes

❑ No

23. Do you feel uncomfortable, anxious or irritated when other people disrupt your rituals or touch your things?

❑ Yes

❑ No

24. Do you feel like your intrusive thoughts and compulsive behaviors have an impact on your life at work, at home or anywhere else?

❑ Yes, a large impact

❑ Yes, a small impact

❑ No impact at all

25. Are you sometimes afraid of losing control of your mind, or acting on one of your impulsions (such as stabbing someone)?

❑ Yes

❑ No

Common difficulties in diagnosis and treatment of OCD

OCD is often accompanied by another disorder such as depression and anxiety. When you suffer from depression, you often have very little motivation or energy and you feel sad. Often, you feel worthless as well. This can delay the diagnosis and treatment of OCD. Your anxiety could cause you to see your symptoms as insurmountable, which in turn could stop you from talking to your doctor.

Sometimes, OCD will cause you to worry about your doctor or your treatment. Several people have reported that their OCD kicked in after they read the side effects list on their medication. They were unable to continue their treatment because they were obsessing over the potential side effects. Others will have a touch of paranoia mixed in with their OCD, causing them to distrust their therapist.

In some cases, the lack of proper resources to treat OCD can be a major obstacle. Some regions do not have an abundance of qualified professionals who practice cognitive behavior therapy (CBT). Other times, patients will see several specialists before finally receiving a diagnosis of OCD. This is due to the fact that health professionals sometimes lack the training to identify OCD symptoms and refer patients for a psychological evaluation.

What you need to remember:
- OCD is very treatable
- Depression and anxiety are also treatable, often with the same medication as OCD
- Seeking treatment is worth it
- You don't have to suffer in silence
- It is possible that your OCD will cause you to doubt or question your treatment, but this is a *symptom of OCD*

- It can take a while before you get a correct diagnosis. Stick with it, as it will give you the best chance of overcoming your disorder.

Once you receive a diagnosis of OCD, your doctor will most likely offer you several treatment options. Usually, the treatment involves cognitive behavior therapy, medication or both. Thousands of people have successfully conquered their OCD symptoms enough to function normally. With the right treatment, you can too.

Chapter 4

*When you change the way you look at things, the things
you look at change.*
—Dr. Wayne Dyer

Different treatment approaches for OCD

In the case of OCD, there is no single treatment that will
work every time. For example, someone who suffers from a
bacterial infection can usually be cured with antibiotics, but
this is not the case for most mental conditions. Conditions
such as OCD require an approach from several different
angles that will work in synergy to balance the person's life.
The combination of different approaches is generally the
most effective route.

One of the most obvious medical treatment options for
OCD involves medication. Today's drugs are very effective
at treating OCD and keeping it under control. However,
they work best when combined with psychotherapy. Even
though medication and therapy seem to be equally effective
in the treatment of OCD, studies suggest that medication

and cognitive behavior therapy together are even more effective than either of the two options separately. Some people like to also add some alternative therapies such as hypnosis and acupuncture. Others find that certain lifestyle changes greatly benefit their OCD treatment. You may have to experiment to find out what works best for you.

The outcome of treatment is different for everyone. Some people find that they receive no benefits from medication and CBT. For the majority, OCD symptoms improve by about 50%, which is often enough to let them have a normal life. Their symptoms no longer prevent them from functioning at work, school and in social situations. Their impulses can be controlled and their anxiety is noticeably lower. For a small percentage of lucky people, medication and/or cognitive behavior therapy brings complete remission from OCD symptoms. In any case, the more effort you invest in your treatment, the more likely you are to see positive results.

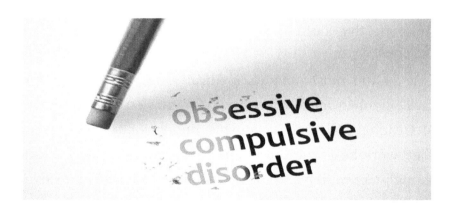

Pharmacological treatment of OCD

While CBT alone is often very effective to treat OCD, some patients benefit from adding a medication to their treatment. There are several reasons behind this:

- Medication alone can reduce the severity of OCD symptoms by 40 to 60% in certain patients, making CBT much more effective.
- Medication can help reduce anxiety, which in turn can make the patient more receptive to CBT.
- OCD is often accompanied by depression. Since the main pharmacological treatments used for OCD are antidepressants, the two conditions are treated with the same medication.

Not all antidepressants are effective in treating OCD. This is because there are various classes of antidepressants which act on different parts of the brain. The most effective medications for OCD are selective serotonin reuptake inhibitors (SSRIs). Because OCD and anxiety are thought to be caused in part by low levels of serotonin, it makes sense that a medication designed to increase the amount of circulating serotonin would have a significant impact on the symptoms.

Serotonin is a neurotransmitter responsible for transmitting information across synapses, the gaps between nerve cells. There are several other neurotransmitters, each with a distinct function. Serotonin is specifically involved in the regulation of appetite, sleep, memory, learning, sexual response, mood and several other biological regulation functions. Patients with low levels of serotonin in their brains tend to exhibit depression and anxiety symptoms, although how exactly this happens is not very well understood yet.

It is not known what role serotonin plays in OCD, but SSRIs are effective in reducing the symptoms associated with the disorder. SSRIs work by selectively preventing serotonin from being recaptured after carrying its message, effectively increasing the amount that is available to transmit impulses across other nearby synapses.

While increasing the levels of serotonin will likely not be enough to treat OCD, it improves the symptoms enough to make people responsive to cognitive behavioral therapy. It can also help lift depression enough to encourage the patient to follow psychotherapy. In short, SSRIs reduce depression, anxiety and OCD symptoms in order to "prepare" the patient for CBT, which is likely to be more effective in those with the right mindset and motivation.

The most common medications to treat OCD are:
- Fluvoxamine (Luvox)
- Paroxetine (Paxil)
- Fluoxetine (Prozac)

- Sertraline (Zoloft)
- Citalopram (Celexa)
- Escitalopram (Lexapro)
- Venlafaxine (Effexor) – This medication belongs to a different class of antidepressants known as SNRIs (serotonin and norepinephrine reuptake inhibitors). It works roughly in the same manner as SSRIs but instead of selectively inhibiting serotonin reuptake, it affects both serotonin and another neurotransmitter known as norepinephrine.
- Clomipramine (Anafranil) – Another "dual action" drug from the SNRI class

There are several other drugs that can be useful in patients who do not respond to the above drugs. For example, duloxetine (Cymbalta) is a new SNRI that provides benefits to certain patients who did not show improvements on SSRIs or older SNRIs.

Antidepressants take a long time to reach their full results. For the first few weeks, you are not very likely to see any positive effects. However, after 10 to 12 weeks, you should notice a marked improvement in your symptoms. Since everybody responds differently to each medication, you may have to try several before you finally find the right one. It is important not to give up on your treatment even if you think it does not provide any benefits. Some people take much longer to respond to SSRIs than others.

All antidepressants should be taken regularly to maintain a constant blood concentration. A sudden drop in the blood concentration of these drugs can trigger unpleasant side effects. Therefore, these treatments are not to be taken on an as-needed basis, unlike benzodiazepines or sleeping pills. Most of them come in tablets or capsules that need to be taken once a day. Skipping a dose will probably not have a significant impact on the treatment as long as it doesn't happen too often. If you forget your dose, just wait until it's time to take your next dose. Do not double up in an attempt to make up for the missed dose.

Side effects

Unfortunately, antidepressants have a rather heavy side effect profile. This does not mean that you shouldn't follow the treatment recommended by your doctor. Many people live successful and happy lives while taking antidepressants. The key is to find the medication that has the greatest benefit with the least side effects in your particular case.

Starting a new antidepressant can be difficult, especially during the first few days. You may suffer from increased anxiety, shaking, dizziness, headaches and nausea. These side effects tend to decrease greatly with time. The most common side effects of antidepressants include:

- Dry mouth
- Blurry vision

- Weight gain
- Insomnia
- Constipation
- Restlessness and anxiety
- Dizziness
- Nausea
- Sexual side effects
- Fatigue
- Increased risk of suicidal thoughts

If these unwanted effects do not decrease after a few weeks of treatment, it could mean you need to switch to a different medication. Sometimes, a different class of antidepressant will be just as effective for your OCD symptoms while causing less undesirable effects.

It should be noted that most antidepressants can increase the risk of suicide in depressed people during the initial weeks of treatment. For this reason, antidepressant treatments should be carefully monitored, even for the treatment of OCD since it is often accompanied by mild to severe depression.

Usually, your doctor will begin a new treatment with small doses and gradually increase to the full dose. This gives your body some time to adapt to a new medication. You may find that the side effects increase a little bit after each dosage increase. This is perfectly normal and the side effects should stabilize after your doctor has found your ideal dose. Generally, your doctor will try to give you the lowest possible dose to limit the side effects. Every medication has the potential to increase the dosage within a certain safe range for people who do not respond to the lowest dose.

Most people who stick to an antidepressant treatment notice a marked improvement in their mood and anxiety levels. These benefits certainly make CBT more effective and increase the likelihood of long-term effects from CBT. So how long should you take your medication in the case of OCD? No one really knows the answer to this question, and it is not the same for everyone. Some people are able to stop all drugs after 6 to 12 months, while at least half will need to be on a low maintenance dose for several years. In some cases, the patient benefits from taking a medication for the rest of his or her life. This all depends on each individual case.

It appears that the risk of relapse is lower in patients who learn CBT techniques while following an effective pharmacological treatment. Once the CBT techniques are acquired and mastered, the medication can be tapered down very slowly, over the course of several months. The techniques that were acquired during psychotherapy often allow patients to control any returning symptoms after medication is discontinued.

Sometimes, symptoms return after a few medication-free weeks or months. Most patients will get a good response if they restart their medication, while others will need to switch to a different one. For this reason, the perspective of stopping a pharmacological treatment should be discussed with your doctor.

OCD medications in children and teens

Currently, the same medications are used for adults, teens and children with OCD. However, only four antidepressants have been approved by the FDA for use in children and teens affected by OCD: clomipramine (Anafranil), fluoxetine (Prozac), fluvoxamine (Luvox) and sertraline (Zoloft). Anafranil is usually not the first choice because of its potential side effects. If necessary, doctors can prescribe other drugs from the SSRI or SNRI class to children.

Usually, children and teens start with very small doses of these drugs and gradually increase it until they reach a full adult-sized dose. OCD often requires these relatively high doses. About 20% of children who take medication for OCD achieved remission (no major OCD symptom), and over 50% of those who combined medication with CBT went into remission. Of those who did not go into remission, a good proportion still showed an improvement of their symptoms.

Cognitive Behavior Therapy (CBT)

CBT is different from traditional psychotherapy. This approach focuses on the problem at hand rather than its roots in your past. The aim of CBT is to change thought patterns in order to elicit a different response from a certain stimulus. For example, if a certain thought causes you to respond in a specific way every time, CBT will help you change the associated response to a different one. CBT is very effective for many people who deal with phobias, anxiety, depression and OCD.

Specifically, the branch of CBT that is used to treat OCD is Exposure and Response Prevention (ERP) therapy. It features a collaborative approach during which you will work with your therapist to conquer the anxiety caused by certain situations.

The "exposure" portion of ERP involves being confronted to the thoughts and objects that drive your OCD and cause your anxiety. The "response prevention" aspect will teach you to overcome the impulse to perform your usual ritual, thus breaking the cycle of OCD. With time, your brain will no longer associate a certain thought to an action that must be accomplished. It teaches your brain to differentiate between real danger and perceived danger by realizing that nothing bad happened as a result of not performing the rituals.

This whole concept can sound scary. However, everything is done under supervision at your own pace. Your therapist will usually start with small steps and work towards bigger goals to help you conquer your obsessive thoughts and compulsive behaviors. Some people have already tried to quit their compulsive behaviors several times, only to find themselves even more anxious. This often drives them to give in and continue performing their rituals, reinforcing the idea that the compulsive behavior must be accomplished in order to reduce anxiety.

In CBT, your therapist will guide you through the steps you need to take in order to successfully detach yourself from the need to perform these compulsive behaviors. For example, if you suffer from the fear of contamination, your therapist might push you to touch an object that you believe is contaminated such as the door handle on a public building. She will then deny you the opportunity to wash your hands for several hours. This forces you to deal with the associated anxiety, which in turn makes you accustomed to these uncomfortable situations. Once your brain realizes that you are not in danger even if you don't wash your hands immediately, your anxiety levels will drop greatly.

For this therapy to be successful, you need to commit to abstaining from performing your compulsive behavior until your levels of anxiety naturally drop. Eventually, you will not even feel the need to perform it at all. You'll realize that everyone else touches door handles and railings on a regular basis without catching all kinds of diseases. Since telling this to your brain in a rational manner does not work, CBT will help you realize it on a subconscious level.

CBT works best if you find a therapist that you trust. Since it can be very emotionally involving, having someone you can trust accompany you during this process can make things much easier. You will work with her to establish objectives that will take you a little further out of your comfort zone every time. Since you will likely go through a lot of anxiety, having a good relationship with your therapist is essential.

After a while, touching "contaminated" objects will no longer trigger an uncontrollable urge to wash your hands because you are now used to it. You saw that nothing happened and it will become increasingly easier to fight the urges until you no longer get them. Some people never fully recover even with CBT and have to deal with a certain level of anxiety every time their OCD is triggered. Usually, with the techniques they learn in CBT, they are still able to overcome this anxiety enough to function in their daily lives.

Your therapist will sometimes give you "homework" to perform outside of the therapy session. An example of an assignment she could give you would be to forego the hand washing after using public transportation. You'd have to hop on a bus, get off somewhere at the park and go for a long walk with your music player. Having something to take your mind off the compulsion will generally help you be more successful.

When you meet with your therapist, it is important to be completely honest with her. If you were unable to perform the assignments she gave you, you need to tell her. She's there to help you and not telling the truth about your progress could ultimately create more anxiety for you as the assignments progress in difficulty.

While ERP is very effective, cognitive behavior therapy also offers another aspect of therapy that can be beneficial for those with OCD. The cognitive aspect of CBT involves changing thought patterns in order to modify your perception of your obsessions. Anxiety is a disproportion between perceived risk and real risk. For example, the chances of starting a fire by leaving an appliance on are extremely slim in reality. The proof is that house fires are very rare and most are caused by malfunctioning equipment, cigarettes and damaged electrical cords/outlets. Chances are, you turned the stove off immediately after you were done using it. For the person with obsessive thoughts about causing a fire by leaving the stove on, the probability of this disaster happening is very high – in their mind. It is often very difficult to differentiate between real and perceived risk.

First, cognitive therapy teaches you to take a step back and evaluate the real risks and consequences involved in a certain situation. Let's look at an example.

Sylvia's story

Sylvia's OCD pushes her to check her alarm clock several dozen times at night. She is afraid of being late for work because she forgot to set her alarm the previous night. In her mind, being late would get her fired, which would lead her to lose her house and her car. She is a single mother of two children, and she fears that she would be an unfit mother if she lost everything. Naturally, this causes a lot of anxiety for Sylvia, who suffers from insomnia. She constantly wakes up during the night to check on her alarm clock, making sure it is plugged in properly, has a spare set of back-up batteries and is set for 6:30 the next morning.

Sylvia consults her doctor because she is exhausted and cannot live like this anymore. She is aware that her obsession with the alarm clock is causing her to lose the precious sleep she needs to perform well at work and take care of her children. Her doctor suggests CBT. During cognitive therapy, Sylvia learns that her mind often makes exaggerated scenarios that it likes to re-run over and over in her mind, causing her to overestimate the actual risks and consequences of a certain situation.

Sylvia's therapist now asks her a few questions:

a. What are the actual chances that you would wake up late for work? How often has it happened in the past?

b. When you woke up to check on your alarm clock, did you ever find out that you had forgotten to set it?

c. What would be the consequences if you were to show up late for work?

d. Would your boss really fire you for missing your alarm clock once?

e. If you really did lose your job, does that mean you would lose your house and car automatically? Are there no other options?

Hopefully, through these questions, Sylvia realizes that the chances of actually forgetting the alarm clock are not very high if she sets it as part of her bedtime routine. She has never forgotten it before and her repeated checking of everything has been essentially useless. She acknowledges that her boss would probably not fire her for a first offense. If she were to be late often enough to lose her job, there are some people around who could help her out while she finds a new job. There are other options such as taking a loan or employment insurance. The chances of losing her house and car are therefore extremely unlikely.

The cognitive therapy process has made Sylvia realize that the scenario she has created is probably never going to happen. She was obsessed with that scenario, which ran over and over in her head. She lost many hours of precious sleep each night worrying about it, which triggered an uncontrollable urge to make sure it wouldn't happen. Her OCD was driven by the fear of being a bad mother if she were to lose her house and her car, which she needs to care for her children.

Sylvia's perceived risks were much higher than the real risks associated with waking up late. In most workplaces, she would receive a verbal warning from her boss. Plenty of people arrive late for work on occasion and it rarely costs them their job. There is therefore an extremely unlikely risk that showing up late at the office one morning would cause her to lose everything. OCD and anxiety often cause people to focus on one possibility while ignoring everything else in between. In Sylvia's case, her anxiety only focuses on the worst possible case, which becomes so real in her mind that she must do everything she can to avoid it.

Of course, this process takes place possibly over several meetings with the therapist, during which Sylvia expresses her concerns. The therapist guides her to draw these conclusions herself. This is essential for effective modification of thought patterns, since what other people tell us is rarely as effective as the things we realize for ourselves.

The second facet of cognitive therapy involves replacing the interpretation of a certain thought by another interpretation. Here is John's story.

John's story
For as long as he can remember, John has suffered from strange thoughts that pop into his head. He frequently has visions of a violent car accident involving his wife and kids. The voice in his head tells him that he is a bad person and doesn't deserve his family. Naturally, John doesn't talk about these things to anybody.

When the horrible thoughts happen, he prays to God in the hopes that He will be gracious enough to grant him another day with his family. He repents himself by picking up the trash on his way to the bus stop or helping his neighbor paint his fence. In fact, he does everything he can to help out other people and feels anxious if he misses an opportunity to lend a hand because God might need to punish him and his family for his laziness.

Normally, John doesn't consider himself a bad person. However, when these thoughts happen, he sees himself as really evil: his family's death would be his fault. If he had been a better person, God wouldn't need to punish his wife and children.

John's compulsive praying and helping others are triggered by thoughts that make him feel guilty. He is terrified that his actions will bring God's wrath upon his family. For this reason, he does everything he can to prove that he is a good person in order to avoid the harm that could come to his loved ones.

Cognitive therapy will guide John through a process that will help him free himself from those thoughts. The belief that his family members' lives depend on the morality of his actions is his own interpretation of the thoughts that come to his mind. Another person could interpret the vision of a car accident differently.

With the help of his therapist, John will learn to challenge this interpretation and attach a new meaning to it. For example, instead of letting the voice tell him that the accident is his fault, he can redirect his thoughts to something else, such as the image of his children playing in the park. The new interpretation attached to the trigger (image of the accident) would be that he cares for his family's safety and well-being.

Over the course of a few therapy sessions, John learns that these images in his mind have the meaning that he has attributed to them. Now, instead of becoming extremely anxious and distressed when he sees the accident, he immediately tells himself how much he loves his family and pictures them playing happily. He is able to control his obsessive need for praying, and he still loves helping out the neighbors but he no longer feels morally obligated to.

For people who follow CBT, a thought journal can help them identify their interpretation of intrusive thoughts, which in turn can facilitate the process of attaching new meanings and interpretations to these thoughts. This thought journal includes information on several aspects in order to help identify patterns and become aware of how your obsessional thoughts behave.

Every time you experience an intrusive thought, write down the following:
1. Where was I and what was I doing when the obsession began?
2. What image/thought came to my mind?
3. What is my interpretation of this thought?
4. How did I respond to it?

The purpose of the thought journal is to write down on paper the things that are happening in your head. This way, you will have an easier time looking at those thoughts objectively and figuring out the thought process behind your compulsions. Your thought journal can be kept to yourself but the better option is to show it to your therapist so she can help you gain insight into your own thought patterns.

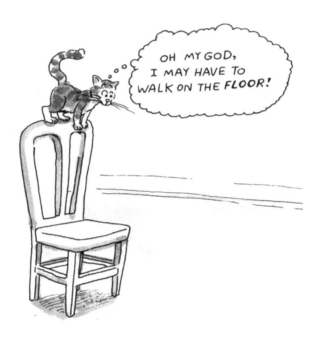

Let's have a look at John's and Sylvia's personal thought journals.

	Sylvia	John
Where am I? What am I doing?	Lying in bed, trying to fall asleep	Watching a football game on TV
What thought came to my mind?	"Did I forget to set my alarm clock?"	Violent image of my family having a car accident
My interpretation	If I forget it, I'll be late for work, lose my job, my house and my car and I'll be an unfit mother.	I'm a bad person and I don't deserve them. I am watching TV while they are running errands. I am crazy for having these recurrent images.
What did I do?	I got up and checked my clock, the batteries, the cord, at least 15 times.	I prayed to God and promised that I would make dinner tonight in order to make up for the time I wasted watching television.

Sylvia and John can now analyze their thought journal entry and try to challenge their thought process. After identifying their thoughts and their interpretations of these thoughts, they need to:

- Find any evidence to support or disprove the obsession.
- Figure out if any cognitive distortions are involved in the thought process.
- Develop an alternative response to the image/thought.

This is the essence of cognitive therapy. CBT that focuses on both the cognitive aspect and ERP is very effective to treat OCD. You'll learn to control your anxiety when exposed to the object of your obsession, you'll learn to break the OCD cycle by resisting the impulse to perform your ritual and you'll learn to challenge your obsessive thoughts in order to attach a new, less threatening meaning to them. These techniques are very simple and effective if you follow your therapist's advice.

Although the principle behind CBT is relatively simple, you should expect the therapy to be difficult. You will be exposed to things that make you anxious in order to teach your brain to differentiate between real and perceived danger. You will have to do your homework, even when it is difficult. Still, thousands of people have successfully used CBT to treat their OCD and they are very happy with the results. The tools you will acquire in a few months of CBT will benefit you for the rest of your life.

Sometimes, CBT is done in a group context because many people with OCD actually feel relieved to meet others who suffer from the same condition. Being able to share experiences and listen to the challenges that others face can be extremely helpful for OCD sufferers, especially those who feel alone.

Serotonin and GABA deficiency diets

While adopting a new diet will not cure OCD, it can improve the symptoms and make them easier to deal with. OCD is sometimes linked with a deficiency in serotonin. Serotonin is a neurotransmitter that is heavily involved in feelings of well-being and happiness. Low levels of this chemical seem to trigger anxiety and depression.

GABA (gamma-amino-butyric acid) is another neurotransmitter that seems to play an important role in mood regulation. Low levels of GABA are consistently found in those with mood and anxiety disorders. While serotonin can be thought of as the "happy" neurotransmitter, GABA can be seen as the "calm" neurotransmitter.

A good balance of chemicals inside the brain is key to a proper regulation of mood and stress. In fact, pharmaceutical drugs work by increasing or decreasing the levels of neurotransmitters inside the brain in order to achieve a certain effect. If you'd rather try a more natural approach, certain foods can help increase the levels of serotonin and GABA.

The happiness diet

This diet is not actually a diet to lose weight. It refers to a specific way of eating that optimizes serotonin and GABA production as well as their efficiency in the brain. Serotonin is made from an amino acid known as L-tryptophan. When your diet doesn't contain enough tryptophan, your body cannot create enough serotonin to balance your mood. The key is to consume tryptophan-rich foods along with some nutrients that help the body convert it to serotonin.

To increase the production of serotonin, try consuming tryptophan-rich foods such as:

- Poultry (especially turkey) – although all meats contain a certain amount of tryptophan, turkey and chicken breast are some of the best sources of this amino acid
- Seafood (especially shrimp)
- Fish (salmon, cod, sardines, tuna, halibut)
- Dairy (milk, cheese, yogurt)
- Nuts and seeds – pumpkin seeds have the highest tryptophan content, followed by cashews, almonds, walnuts and sunflower seeds
- Tofu and soy milk

- Legumes – kidney and black beans are at the top of the legume list, followed by peanuts
- Grains (oats, wheat, corn, brown rice, barley)
- Fruits such as bananas and dates

You'll notice that most of the tryptophan-rich foods are excellent sources of protein. This is because proteins are made up of amino acids, which can be thought of as the "building blocks" of proteins. A good rule of thumb is to eat plenty of protein-rich foods in order to boost levels of serotonin in the brain.

Eating tryptophan-rich foods, however, will not be enough to increase the levels of serotonin in the brain. To create neurotransmitters, the body needs several other nutrients. Complex carbohydrates are necessary to trigger the reaction that causes the brain to synthetize serotonin from tryptophan. Good sources of complex carbohydrates include:

- Fruits such as bananas, apples, figs, pineapple, kiwis
- Whole grains such as brown rice, oats, corn, quinoa and kamut
- Vegetables such as potatoes, spinach, carrots, broccoli
- Legumes such as dry beans and peas

Other vitamins and minerals are also essential to make serotonin. Vitamins from the B-complex, vitamin C and magnesium are among the most important ones. These vitamins and minerals can be found in:

- Leafy greens
- Tofu
- Eggs
- Seeds
- Brown rice and corn
- Citrus fruit and bananas

Omega-3 fatty acids also contribute to increase the levels of serotonin in the brain. These essential fatty acids are found in oily seeds, nuts and fish such as:

- Walnuts
- Hemp, chia and flax seeds
- Fatty fish such as salmon, mackerel, anchovies, sardines

A good balance of these nutrients is necessary to increase the production of serotonin in the brain. If one of the elements is missing in the chain, serotonin production will not be optimal. Some nutrients are necessary to absorb other nutrients while some trigger chemical reactions. They are all equally important and a successful serotonin- and GABA-boosting diet includes a variety of healthy foods such as those listed above.

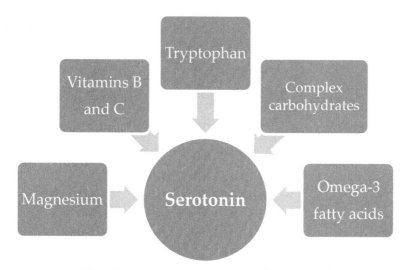

The dietary components of serotonin

Foods to avoid

Caffeinated drinks can seem great for a temporary energy boost, but they deplete serotonin levels. Drinking green tea or herbal tea can be a better alternative. Although green tea contains some caffeine, its content is much lower than coffee. As a bonus, green tea contains another nutrient that can help with OCD: L-theanine.

Avoid anything too refined such as candy, sugary drinks, white bread and pasta, chips and other nutrient-poor foods. The key when trying to balance neurotransmitters is to eat fresh, nutrient-rich foods to give the body the nutrition it needs to build serotonin, GABA and other important chemicals.

Avoid alcohol. It temporarily increases the release of serotonin, which causes the characteristic happy feeling that you get after a few drinks. However, once the high wears off, serotonin levels are depleted. The lower serotonin levels are, the higher the risk of depression and anxiety. This is also true for most stimulant drugs, which have devastating effects on serotonin supplies.

GABA boosters

GABA is available in supplement form but it is very inefficient when delivered orally. Sometimes, your best bet is to increase production by consuming certain foods. GABA is made from a combination of the amino acid glutamine and vitamin B6 (pyridoxine). As a result, consuming foods that contain these two nutrients can help increase GABA levels. Some of these foods include:

- Organ meats (liver, kidney)
- Fish
- Brown rice, wheat and oats
- Lentils and beans
- Cantaloupe, oranges and other fresh citrus, mushrooms
- Broccoli
- Turkey and beef
- Almonds, walnuts

Conveniently, many foods that are rich in tryptophan also help regulate GABA levels. The ideal serotonin and GABA deficiency diet focuses on lean meats such as turkey and chicken, liver, fish, whole grains, legumes, tofu, dairy and colorful fruits and veggies (bananas, citrus, leafy greens, etc.) Some nuts, seeds and eggs make great additions as well. Consuming these foods on a daily basis will provide a healthy dose of serotonin- and GABA-building nutrients.

Other nutrients can also assist in the production of GABA. As mentioned earlier, green tea contains L-theanine, which helps with the production of GABA. L-theanine is also found in nuts, spinach, oats and whole grains. B-vitamins, which help with energy metabolism, and minerals such as calcium and magnesium are also essential to synthetize GABA.

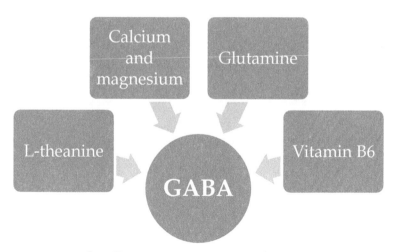

The dietary components of GABA

Herbal teas that stimulate GABA and serotonin production
While not technically herbal, green tea's L-theanine produces a calming effect on the brain and increases levels of serotonin, dopamine and GABA.

Passionflower and valerian are two well-known herbs that help with anxiety and insomnia. They are often combined in teas along with lemon balm and other calming herbs. These herbal mixes, sometimes known as "good night" teas, are believed to have a calming effect by elevating GABA levels.

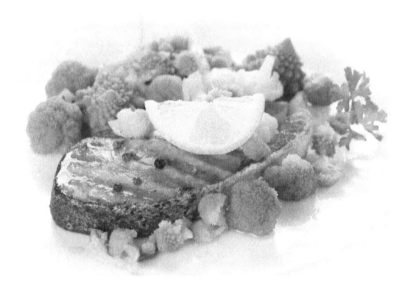

Summary of serotonin and GABA deficiency diet		
Poultry	Vitamin B	Serotonin, GABA
(chicken, turkey)	Tryptophan	Serotonin
	Glutamine	GABA
Liver	Glutamine	GABA
Legumes	Complex carbs	Serotonin
(dried beans,	Tryptophan	Serotonin
lentils, tofu)	Glutamine	GABA
Dairy	Tryptophan	Serotonin
(yogurt, cheese)	Calcium	GABA
Fish	Glutamine	GABA
(mackerel,	Omega-3	Serotonin
sardines, salmon)	Tryptophan	Serotonin
Whole grains	Complex carbs	Serotonin
(wheat, oats, corn,	Tryptophan	Serotonin
brown rice)	Glutamine	GABA
	Vitamin B	Serotonin, GABA
	L-theanine	Serotonin, GABA
Seeds	Omega-3	Serotonin
(hemp, chia, flax)	Vitamin B	Serotonin, GABA
Starchy veggies	Complex carbs	Serotonin
(potatoes)	Vitamin C	Serotonin
Leafy greens	Vitamin C	Serotonin
(spinach, swiss	Magnesium	Serotonin
chard, kale)	Complex carbs	Serotonin
Nuts	Omega-3	Serotonin
(almonds,	Tryptophan	Serotonin
walnuts)	L-theanine	Serotonin, GABA
Fruits	Complex carbs	Serotonin
(bananas, dried	Magnesium	Serotonin, GABA
dates, figs, melons,	Vitamin B	Serotonin, GABA
citrus)	Vitamin C	Serotonin

This chart summarizes the most "efficient" foods when trying to rebalance the brain chemicals involved in OCD. Of course, every natural food contains something good that can benefit the body, but the above list will provide the best value when aiming for serotonin and GABA balance. At least one or two foods from this list should be included in every meal, with a good variety throughout the day.

Physical activity

Physical exercise can help improve your sense of well-being. Many studies highlight the benefits of exercise as a natural and healthy way to decrease anxiety, improve the quality of sleep, elevate mood and increase self-esteem. Physical exercise stimulates the release of several brain chemicals such as serotonin and endorphins. Serotonin makes you feel happier and endorphins act like natural painkillers. Both these chemicals reduce stress and make you feel good.

Exercise can also improve alertness, concentration and energy levels. If your OCD makes it difficult to concentrate or sleep when all kinds of thoughts invade your mind, you may find that engaging in moderate physical activity will help you greatly in those aspects. Since OCD is an anxiety disorder, reducing stress and improving the quality of sleep can certainly be beneficial, especially when combined with a healthy diet.

Although any type of physical activity can be beneficial, yoga may hold a special place in the treatment of OCD. Yoga involves a full-body approach that takes care of the physical and spiritual aspects of the person. Since yoga combines specific movements known as "poses" with breathing exercises and meditation, it is excellent as a de-stressor. The poses gently stretch your muscles, the breathing exercises help you relax and distract you from your obsessions, and the meditation exercises encourage you to learn how to clear your mind.

Herbal supplements

While they can be very useful, natural herbal supplements should be used with caution. They are not regulated by government agencies such as the FDA or Health Canada, meaning the quality and concentration of the product can vary greatly between different manufacturers. They can also interact with prescribed medication, so you should always talk to your doctor if you are considering the use of herbal supplements.

A wide variety of natural products can be used to treat anxiety disorders. Some of them help you relax while others boost the production of serotonin, GABA and other brain chemicals. Here is a list of some popular herbal remedies that can have benefits for people with OCD. Keep in mind that most of these supplements have no scientifically proven benefits and should be used as alternative therapies when conventional treatments don't work because of a lack of response or severe side effects. Some people have had success with these supplements but they may not work for everyone.

St. John's Wort

This supplement, made from the flowers and leaves of an herb, has proven benefits for those who suffer from mild to moderate depression. There are several other indications for this product, but the scientific evidence is still not very strong. In the case of OCD, the scientific community is on the fence about St. John's Wort. Some studies have shown some benefits while other studies have not found any. In any case, since OCD is often accompanied by depressive symptoms, St. John's Wort could be useful to help with these symptoms.

If you are considering the use of St. John's Wort for OCD, depression and anxiety, talk to your doctor first. It has many potential drug interactions, namely with antidepressants, pain relievers and anti-anxiety medications. Your doctor will be able to recommend a dosage and review your current medication to make sure you will not suffer from a dangerous drug interaction.

Inositol

Inositol is a vitamin from the B-complex. According to research, it breaks down into two different chemicals that enhance the action of serotonin in the brain. Although strong scientific evidence of the usefulness of inositol to reduce OCD symptoms is still lacking, several case studies have had success with their patients. Inositol is not usually a first-line treatment, but it is rather used in patients who do not respond to antidepressant medications, or who need to discontinue such medications because of side effects. It can be used on its own, or in combination with antidepressants.

5-HTP

5-hydroxy-L-tryptophan (5-HTP) is an immediate precursor to serotonin. It is naturally synthesized from tryptophan, but it can also be taken in supplement form. Although it has proven benefits for depression and anxiety, the evidence of its usefulness in the treatment of OCD is once again mixed. Since 5-HTP transforms into serotonin, it needs to be used under medical supervision. Too much serotonin puts you at risk for a dangerous condition known as *serotonin syndrome.* It should not be used with antidepressants or St. John's Wort.

L-tryptophan

L-tryptophan is an essential amino acid that plays a role in the production of serotonin. Since drugs that modify the release or the reuptake of serotonin have proven benefits for OCD, some studies were conducted on the potential benefits of L-tryptophan. Although more evidence is needed, preliminary studies have found that 6 grams of L-tryptophan successfully reduced OCD symptoms in subjects. L-tryptophan can also consumed in protein-rich foods. In fact, diet would be the better approach since the body is very inefficient at absorbing supplement forms of L-tryptophan.

L-theanine

L-theanine is found in green tea and a few other foods. Anecdotal evidence reports some benefits in the treatment of OCD, although more serious research is needed on the subject. L-theanine increases alertness and reduces anxiety, presumably by increasing the levels of GABA. Supplements of L-theanine can benefit some people by reducing their anxiety levels and improving their ability to concentrate on tasks.

Passionflower

Passionflower is a gentle relaxant. Once again, no definitive research has concluded that passionflower has clear benefits in the treatment of OCD, but some people have had success with it. Decreasing anxiety levels associated with intrusive thoughts and increasing the quality of sleep can have beneficial effects for those who suffer from OCD. Some studies suggest that it has a minor effect on the regulation of serotonin reuptake in the brain, potentially lowering OCD symptoms.

Alternative therapies

Hypnosis and NLP

Hypnosis and neuro linguistic programming (NLP) are widely used in the treatment of mental conditions. These techniques focus on reaching the subconscious through suggestions, allowing you to change your though patterns. Both techniques have had spectacular results on some people suffering from various ailments.

Since OCD is made up of repetitive patterns (the same thought triggers the same behavior every time), simply altering these patterns can contribute to free someone from obsessions and compulsions. NLP acts on the conscious mind while hypnosis reaches the unconscious mind. Either can be used separately, or they can be used together to increase effectiveness. NLP works on helping you distinguish real danger from perceived danger while hypnosis helps you change your interpretation and automatic response to certain stimuli (obsessive ideas).

NLP and hypnosis work very well when performed by specialists. However, the sessions are usually expensive and don't work for everyone. A small percentage of people cannot be hypnotized, and another percentage of the population is either scared of hypnosis or doesn't really believe in it.

Some self-hypnosis sessions are available for free or for a small fee on the Internet. These sessions can be helpful but they are not tailored to your specific needs. Nevertheless, some people have had success in reducing their symptoms by using the self-help hypnotherapy sessions. They require dedication and concentration, but they are very safe, meaning you can try them a few times to see if this type of solution could work for you.

Acupuncture
Acupuncture is a form of ancient traditional Chinese medicine. Tiny needles are inserted in different "points" throughout the body to rebalance the energy flow. Some people have had success using this form of alternative therapy for their anxiety disorder. However, this method may not work for everyone. It is based on thousands of years of practice rather than scientific evidence.

According to ancient Chinese medicine, anxiety is caused by an imbalance in the energy flow between the kidneys and the heart. Acupuncture attempts to correct this imbalance. Obviously, the effectiveness of acupuncture depends partially on your view of the ancient Chinese conception of health, relating different conditions to the energy flow in organs. However, acupuncture has been recognized as a legitimate treatment for some conditions by Western medicine, and many people resort to this natural option in the hopes of obtaining relief from their symptoms.

General tips on dealing with obsessive thoughts

When you feel the urge to perform your ritual, it often helps to do something that takes your mind off the compulsion for several minutes. It delays the compulsive response and your brain does not associate it as strongly with the obsession. For example, if you feel the urge to go wash your hands, you could call your mother, go for a jog, listen to your favorite song, read a book or play with your pet. The idea is to shift your attention from your obsession to something you enjoy. Ideally, you will work towards delaying the impulse long enough that it will go away on its own.

Many people like to tell themselves when they are having an obsessive thought. If you always check on appliances and locks repeatedly, you can learn to tell yourself "This is my OCD. I have already checked the door and it was locked. All the appliances are off. These thoughts are a symptom of my OCD." Tell yourself that you are closing the window while you are doing it. It will help you make the connection between the action and the result.

Save your worries for a specific period during the day. Every time an anxious thought comes to your mind, tell yourself that you will deal with it later during the "worry period". Allow 5 or 10 minutes each day, preferably always in the same place at the same time, and let your mind run its course. The worry period is there for your mind to express your anxiety. You should not try to rationalize or stop the negative thoughts. Once the worry period is over, you can take a few minutes to relax, do some breathing exercises and go back to your activities. The rest of the day is designated as worry-free.

Train yourself to ignore the signals from the OCD brain circuit. You know what your obsessions are, and you know the rituals you perform in response. When obsessive thoughts happen, you can learn to tell yourself "This thought has no meaning. It is created by my brain to get me to do something I don't want to do. This is a false message from my brain, and I am not in danger. I can safely ignore it."

Helping a loved one with OCD

There are several guidelines when dealing with a loved one who suffers from OCD. As we have seen throughout this book, OCD is not rational. You can't just "snap out of it" and your loved one will not eventually "grow out of it". It is a complex condition brought on by a combination of biological, environmental and lifestyle factors, with a little bit of emotional and social factors thrown in. To really help your family member or friend who suffers from OCD, follow these general guidelines:

- **Avoid criticizing their behavior.** If they repeat certain questions or behaviors, they are probably very aware and ashamed of it.

- **Don't punish a child's OCD behaviors.** They are symptoms caused by a medical condition. The added pressure from the fear of punishment could make things worse.

- **Be kind and patient.** People with OCD often feel crazy, alone and misunderstood. They need someone who doesn't judge them. They need to go through the process of conquering OCD at their own pace. Focus on their progress and share their victories.

- **Do not let yourself be involved in OCD rituals.** If a loved one's OCD tries to involve you, kindly refuse and explain your reasons. Playing along will reinforce their obsessive thoughts. Make sure you give the person your full support and availability while making it clear that you cannot be a part of the rituals.

- **Don't let OCD become the focus of family life.** OCD is a medical condition that can cause some frictions within a family, but it should not be allowed to take over. Try to talk about things other than OCD behaviors. Make family life as normal and stress-free as possible.

- **Focus on communication**. Sometimes, a loved one with OCD will need an honest opinion. You need to find the balance between sugar-coating your words and saying something that could cause distress. Being honest, using proven communication techniques and acting out of kindness should help guide your actions.

- **Laugh**. OCD can be funny at times. If your loved one can find the humor in a situation, it will help provide some relief to the tension that can result from OCD. Of course, this only works if the person affected by OCD finds it funny too.

Living with someone who has OCD can be frustrating at times. However, you need to remember that they are going through something very difficult. Who knows how any of us would react in their situation! Each one of us is different and we each have our worries, our qualities, our talents and our "kind of annoying" characteristics. OCD is a medical condition just like diabetes and cancer. The behaviors are certainly not performed with the goal to annoy people around. They are the person's only means of dealing with anxiety.

Remember:
- They are not usually happy with their condition.

- They cannot control their thoughts and impulsions.
- They have to deal with horrific thoughts and images.
- They feel guilty and responsible for everything.
- Their rituals are often done with the goal of protecting their loved ones.
- They are usually ashamed of their behaviors and have tried many times to stop doing them.

Openly showing your frustration will cause more anxiety for your loved one. Learning about the condition and being genuinely helpful will likely benefit him or her more than punishment or ultimatums. It is nobody's fault that your child, sibling, parent of friend developed OCD, and in most cases they would definitely seize the opportunity if they could just "get rid of it". OCD is a daily challenge for those who live with it, as well as their loved ones. Learning how to deal with this challenge together will maximize the chances of success.

Using OCD to your advantage

Having OCD certainly sucks, but sometimes we have to make the best out of the cards we were dealt. Some people have found creative ways to use their obsessive compulsive disorder to their advantage. Even if treatment will often allow you to live a normal life, you will likely continue to deal with some forms of obsessive thoughts and compulsions.

Having mild OCD can actually benefit you in several ways. You are prone to developing routines, which means you are less likely to forget to do regular things such as taking medication, watering the plants or paying the bills. If you have a tendency to make lists, use that to your advantage by keeping organized lists of tasks, appointments and meetings. You will soon realize that you are not likely to forget as many things as other people, making you reliable and dependable.

Creating a detailed shopping list can help you save money at the grocery store. Maybe you enjoy creating menus for the week, ensuring that you get adequate nutrition and even saving you money since you don't have to order take-out as often. Your house is likely to be more organized; you won't have to waste time looking for your keys or the screwdriver since you already know where everything is.

Some people have found that OCD gave them the focus they needed to finish a certain project. For example, their obsessive nature causes them to work on that task until it is finished. This particular talent is useful for those who write books or participate in projects that require a lot of work. They describe it as a certain mindset that can give them an edge over other people who sometimes get discouraged halfway through a project.

People with OCD often have several strong qualities that can be invaluable in certain jobs. For example, a position as consultant in a large company requires methodical thinking, the ability to plan everything down to the last detail, the ability to make very rational decisions, the ability to avoid taking unnecessary risks and the desire to get things done. These qualities are often found in those with OCD, making them perfect candidates for these positions.

Some jobs are really well-suited for people with OCD, whether they utilize their particular attention to detail or their ability to work alone for extended periods of time. Obviously, you need to find a job that interests you and puts your talents to good use. For some ideas, here is a short list of careers that tend to work well with OCD:

- Accountant: Working with numbers, performing repetitive tasks that require concentration and attention to detail could be perfect for you. Accounting requires motivated, self-driven individuals who aren't afraid of routine work.
- Librarian: This type of job is fairly relaxed, allowing you plenty of time for interaction with customers. It definitely puts your organizational skills to good use.
- Computer Software Engineer: This job requires meticulous attention to detail as well as the ability to check and recheck your work. This can work well with someone who suffers from OCD.

- Quality control: This job is all about making sure that certain products or services are delivered according to specific quality standards. As long as the standards are clear and that there are no gray areas, someone with mild OCD is likely to excel at this work.

- Online customer support agent: This job generally offers flexible hours and allows you to walk away from the keyboard if your anxiety reaches high levels. You'll have no direct interaction with customers, which can be an advantage for some people.

When choosing a career, try to find something that doesn't involve high levels of stress or anxiety. For example, while nursing can certainly benefit from some of the OCD qualities, it is a very stressful job with long hours which might not be suited for someone who suffers from an anxiety disorder. Any relatively low-stress job that utilizes your skills and talents can be a potentially great match. Having a job that you enjoy and that you are good at can certainly help lower your anxiety and increase your self-esteem.

Essentially, once you accept your OCD, it will become much easier to find the perks of having the disorder and use them to your advantage.

Chapter 5

Questions and answers about OCD

Even after reading this book, you probably still have some questions about OCD and its treatment. This section is meant to answer some common questions in a clear, concise manner. Any additional questions that you may have can be answered by your doctor.

How do I really know if I have OCD?
There is no better way to tell if you have OCD than by going through the diagnosis process. Unfortunately, there is no simple blood test or brain scan that can confirm an OCD diagnosis. Only a qualified professional can do a proper psychological evaluation and confirm that you are affected by OCD. Self-tests and other tools are designed to help you identify whether you have any OCD symptoms and how much they affect you in order to seek professional help if necessary.

Are things like compulsive self-harm considered OCD behaviors?
The causes of self-harm are usually not linked with the causes of OCD behaviors. Self-harm is often done when you feel emotionally empty or when emotional pain is so great that you need a physical outlet to express it. OCD compulsions are derived from an intrusive though that triggers anxiety. In other words, self-harm is not usually done with the goal of relieving anxiety but rather to relieve deep emotional pain or numbness. For the purposes of establishing a diagnosis, self-harm behaviors are not generally taken into account.

However, some compulsive self-harm behaviors can be done in a context of OCD. For example, someone who suffers from major depression along with OCD can often have self-harm and suicidal behaviors. Sometimes, the compulsion caused by anxiety can involve self-harm: if your intrusive thought causes you to believe you're a bad person, maybe your compulsion will be to punish yourself by self-harming. These cases are not very common.

Am I at risk of acting on some of my horrific thoughts?
OCD will sometimes cause you to have recurrent images or impulses of very violent things involving inappropriate sexual thoughts, cannibalism or homicide. While very disturbing, these thoughts are symptoms of the condition. If these thoughts are caused by OCD, you are no more likely to act on them than anyone else. Many people who are

plagued with these thoughts are afraid of losing control and acting on their impulses but you can reassure yourself: this does not happen in the case of OCD.

Most of the time, people with OCD who experience these recurring disturbing thoughts see them as separate from themselves. In other words, the action is not performed by who they really are, but by who they are afraid of being. Compulsions will not be geared towards acting out these thoughts but towards neutralizing the obsession and making sure that no one was hurt. It's like being afraid that a monster lives inside you and pushes you to do horrible things, even if you know that you would never do these things. You try to keep the monster under control and prevent any harm it could do.

Can OCD symptoms be related to another condition?
Many conditions share some symptoms with OCD. In fact, OCD symptoms are often mistaken for depression, bipolar disorder, general anxiety disorder or schizophrenia. These other mental conditions can also co-occur with OCD, making diagnosis a very complex process. Also, distinguishing OCD from OCPD (obsessional compulsive personality disorder) can be very hard. Your doctor will often look at what drives your symptoms in order to be able to pinpoint their source.

For example, if your main symptom is cleaning your house, your therapist will need to figure out the thought process behind the action. If you spend hours cleaning your house because you strive for perfection, it's more likely that you suffer from OCPD. If you have gotten a sudden regain of energy after a depressive episode and you are planning all kinds of grandiose things that you prepare for by scrubbing everything until it is perfectly clean, it could be an indication of bipolar disorder. If you clean everything because germs could hide anywhere and you are afraid that your family will get sick, OCD is most likely the cause.

What is the relationship between OCD, anxiety and depression?
These three conditions frequently appear with each other. Approximately 75% of people affected by OCD also suffer from depression. More often than not, depression is also accompanied by anxiety. Depression and anxiety fuel each other, and if you add OCD in the mix, it could certainly affect the condition's outcome. Fortunately, anxiety, depression and OCD are treated with the same type of medications and the same type of psychotherapy (CBT), meaning you can effectively overcome all these conditions with a single treatment plan.

OCD is often hard to detect because the symptoms are hidden by depressive or anxiety symptoms. Once again, the only way to know is to proceed to a complete psychological examination of your thoughts, behaviors and the patterns that fuel these behaviors.

What's the difference between recurring thoughts caused by depression and OCD obsessions?

The morbid thoughts caused by depression, sometimes known as ruminations, often have your sense of self-worth as the central theme. You worry about things that are important to most people, such as your accomplishments in life, your ability to succeed in your projects and your relationships with others. These thoughts are often tainted with regrets. Depressive ruminations tend to be about the past while OCD obsessions are usually about the present or the future, specifically to avoid disasters.

What is the difference between worries caused by anxiety and OCD obsessions?

The distinction often lies in the contents of the thoughts as well as the presence or the absence of anxiety-relieving compulsions. Anxiety will cause you to worry about your performance at school or at work, finances, relationship issues or a sick relative. OCD obsessions will have you focus on something often unrealistic such as the possibility that your family will die if you don't get dressed in a specific order.

In both cases, the anxiety caused by the anticipated situation is excessive. For example, the anxious person will worry excessively about money, causing insomnia, recurring thoughts and possibly panic attacks. The OCD person will also worry excessively about money, but instead of having a panic attack, he or she will perform a ritual in order to avoid a possible financial disaster. The triggering thought is the same, but the thought process and reaction is different.

Will my OCD trigger panic attacks?
In OCD, panic attacks are generally caused by an extreme fear of something. For someone with a panic attack disorder, a stressful situation can trigger a panic attack, which can be thought of as being afraid of being afraid. In OCD, anxious thoughts will not trigger a panic attack since the compulsion exists to relieve extreme anxiety. However, if a person with contamination OCD comes in contact with something soiled by bodily fluids (for example, a drunk person vomits on them), then the panic attack can be triggered because the compulsion can no longer prevent contamination, which has already occurred.

What is normal checking behavior versus compulsive (pathological) checking behavior?
OCD behaviors become problematic when they interfere with your daily life. If you have a strange compulsive routine before leaving the house (check all windows exactly twice, check appliances three times and check the locks five times) but that this routine otherwise does not consume any

more of your time, it is not OCD. It becomes pathological when it consumes great amounts of time (more than one hour per day) or interferes with your daily life (you miss an appointment because you were checking doors and locks for half an hour).

What results can I expect from medication and therapy?
According to the Brain and Behavior Foundation, SSRIs successfully reduce OCD symptoms in 40 to 60% of patients. Those who respond to medication can expect a 40 to 60% decrease in symptoms while those who respond well to CBT can expect closer to a 60 to 80% reduction in their symptoms. These improvements are significant since they often make the difference between severe and moderate or mild OCD. Severe OCD is debilitating, and improving symptoms by 40 to 80% can contribute to give the person the opportunity to function normally at work, at school and at home with minimal management of anxiety when necessary.

What is the most effective treatment for OCD?
As we saw above, CBT usually yields the best results in term of symptom reduction. However, patients are not always ready to undertake CBT, especially is they suffer from depression. If this is your case, your doctor will often choose to prescribe an SSRI for a certain period of time (a few months to a year or more) in order to stabilize your mood and give you the necessary motivation to go through

CBT. Since CBT is most effective in those who are very motivated, adding a medication can sometimes be the better choice.

Will I have to take an SSRI for life?
Some people need to continue taking medications for life while other can be successfully weaned off after a certain period of time. It all depends on your individual response to CBT and medication. If discontinuing your medication results in the return of symptoms, you will probably need to start taking it again. Symptoms usually take a few weeks to return after stopping your medication. In this case, restarting your medication should fix the problem. If you see no return of symptoms, chances are that you will be able to stay off the medications and apply CBT techniques to deal with the occasional anxiety.

Do other people get obsessions and/or compulsions?
A 2010 survey indicated that as much as 28% of the population suffers from obsessions and/or compulsions. However, in most of these cases, they are not pathological (meaning they have no significant impact on the person's life). When you have OCD, your obsessions and compulsions are often (but not always) related to each other and they occupy much of your time or cause you significant distress.

A minor compulsion such as the need to wear green socks on Monday will not disrupt your daily life unless you spend an hour thinking about how wearing those green socks on Monday will prevent someone from dying. If you can't find your green socks Monday morning, how will you react? If you're simply upset but you move on, it's not OCD. If you are genuinely terrified that you have just sparked something terrible, it is probably OCD.

Obsessions and compulsions can also be pathological without being OCD. Compulsive gambling, shopping and playing are more like addictions. They are not caused by anxiety but rather by seeking a specific emotion (excitement, etc.) Obsessing over someone can fuel jealousy, violence and other destructive behaviors, but it is not OCD.

Are people with OCD aware that their thoughts and behaviors are irrational?
Often, they are very aware of that fact, leading to shame, embarrassment and isolation. People with OCD are often very rational and they are plagued by irrational thoughts that cause them to perform irrational actions. This contributes to the distressing aspect of OCD.

In people with OCD, insight will not help lower the anxiety caused by intrusive thoughts. The anxiety will only be relieved (temporarily) by performing a ritual. This ritual can seem silly even for the person doing it. They know they have checked the appliances 17 times already, but they will not feel better until they check again, and again. They are usually unable to explain how this ritual makes them feel better. They just know they have to do it.

Some people have no insight on their condition. They really believe all the thoughts that go through their head. In children, this is more common since they don't yet have the ability to distinguish between real and made-up thoughts.

What is the difference between a normal "neat freak" or "germaphobe" and someone with OCD?
A "neat freak" likes things clean and orderly. It is not OCD if it is part of your personality. If you realize that your concern for neatness or contamination is excessive and that you have tried many times to stop obsessing over these thoughts, it could be related to OCD. Many people will carry a bottle of sanitizer in their purse and use it often. They are a little bit afraid of germs and try to lower their risk of catching something by practicing personal hygiene. This is normal as long as it doesn't have any consequences on their lives.

Why can't people with OCD just stop performing their rituals?
Having OCD is sometimes described as a "broken record". Something in your brain is stuck on a certain idea and it will be repeated over and over again. Just like the record will likely not start playing properly on its own, the

symptoms of OCD will not usually improve without some outside help. Telling someone to stop washing their hands or checking the locks will be useless, since they already know it is excessive. Chances are, focusing on their behavior by disapproving or scolding will cause more anxiety and fuel the OCD cycle.

Will I always have the same obsessions and compulsions?
Symptoms often change over time, especially in children. Someone with contamination OCD can suddenly switch to checking symptoms or compulsive hoarding. There is no way to predict these switches in symptoms, and the best way to deal with them is by treating the cause. Sometimes, new obsessions and compulsions will appear, while other times they will just replace the old ones. CBT and medication help deal with the anxiety behind the behavior, so the behavior does not need to happen, no matter what it.

Is it my fault that my child has OCD?
Although OCD has a genetic component, it is nobody's fault that someone develops OCD or another mental disorder. Some people have genetic predispositions that are triggered by certain events or certain infections. Others will develop OCD for no apparent reason. Nobody is safe from illness, whether physical or mental, and it is certainly not your fault that your child has OCD. You are not responsible for hidden genes that were passed on to your children, and feeling guilty will not change anything. The best way to

deal with a child who has OCD is to support him or her throughout the diagnosis and treatment process, which can be quite scary for a young child. Having Mom's and/or Dad's full support is invaluable for a child going through something like that.

How is OCD severity measured?

Several scales, such as the Yale-Brown Obsessive Compulsive Scale, can help your doctor determine the severity of your symptoms by evaluating their impact on your life, the amount of distress they cause you and how much control you have over them.

Are medications other than SSRIs sometimes used to treat OCD?

SSRIs are most effective at treating OCD symptoms. However, OCD is often accompanied by another disorder which requires a different medication. Some specific symptoms of OCD can also require medication. For example, someone who experiences high anxiety and panic attacks along with OCD could benefit from anxiety medications such as benzodiazepines, which act on the GABA system to quickly and effectively reduce anxiety. Someone who suffers from insomnia as a result of OCD could be prescribed some sleep aids such as benzodiazepines, trazodone or zopiclone.

Secondary medications can be used to increase the effectiveness of an SSRI. Adding an antipsychotic or buspirone to an SSRI can sometimes have modest benefits on OCD symptoms. However, these benefits are not proven and these secondary medications often have a relatively heavy side effect profile. They should be used with caution.

What should I do to help myself during treatment?
Your doctor will be able to suggest some ways in which you can help yourself. Practicing the concepts you learn in CBT and doing your homework are definitely great strategies. Taking your medication as prescribed will also increase the chances of success. General lifestyle changes can help you lower your anxiety. Find a low-stress job that you like. Eat healthy serotonin- and GABA-enhancing foods (see chapter 4 for more information), engage in some physical activity, establish a regular sleep pattern and make time for social activities.

Some self-help books can reinforce the concepts you learn in CBT and generally help you develop an awareness of your capabilities and how to use them. Stay away from drugs and alcohol, at least in excessive amounts. An occasional glass of wine won't hurt, but using alcohol and drugs to cope with stress is not a healthy strategy. Get some sunlight to help with depressive symptoms. Finally, and importantly, have some hope: OCD can be conquered!

Conclusion

Whether you live with OCD yourself or one of your loved ones is affected by it, seeking more information about the condition will make it easier to cope. With the powerful tools from cognitive behavior therapy, you will eventually develop your own strategies to help you deal with anxiety. There is no universal treatment because each person is unique. An approach tailored to your specific needs will greatly help you overcome this often debilitating condition.

The more time and effort you invest in your treatment, the more likely you are to succeed at freeing yourself from the limits imposed by your medical condition. You will become comfortable at dealing with anxiety and you will even learn to use your OCD traits to your advantage. At this point, you will truly have triumphed over your illness.

References

"Acupuncture, Anxiety and Depression." PsychCentral.
http://psychcentral.com/lib/acupuncture-anxiety-depression/00017321

"Antidepressants: Get Tips to Cope With Side Effects."
Mayo Clinic.
http://www.mayoclinic.org/diseases-conditions/depression/in-depth/antidepressants/art-20049305?pg=1

"Anxiety Disorders." National Institute of Mental Health.
http://www.nimh.nih.gov/health/publications/anxiety-disorders/index.shtml?wvsessionid=wv650bd43245ce40588
4dd789794894544

"Careers for People With OCD." Love To Know Jobs and Careers.
http://jobs.lovetoknow.com/careers-people-ocd

"Causes of OCD." Anxiety Care UK.
http://www.anxietycare.org.uk/docs/ocdcauses.asp

"Cognitive Behavior Therapy (CBT)." International OCD Foundation.
http://www.ocfoundation.org/cbt.aspx

"Compulsive Symptoms can be resolved with hypnosis, hypnotherapy and pure hypnoanalysis." International Association of Pure Hypnoanalysts.
http://www.iaph.org/symptoms_treated/compulsive_sympt oms.htm

"Depression." OCD-UK.
http://www.ocduk.org/depression

"Frequently Asked Questions." The Gateway Institute.
http://www.gatewayocd.com/faq.htm

"Frequently Asked Questions About Obsessive-Compulsive Disorder." Brain and Behavior Research Foundation.
http://bbrfoundation.org/frequently-asked-questions-about-obsessive-compulsive-disorder-ocd

"Frequently Asked Questions About OCD." PsychCentral.
http://psychcentral.com/lib/frequently-asked-questions-about-ocd/000502

"Frequently Asked Questions About OCD." Yale School of Medicine: OCD Research Clinic.
http://psychiatry.yale.edu/ocd/patients/ocdfaq.aspx

"History of OCD." Stanford School of Medicine.
http://ocd.stanford.edu/treatment/history.html

"How Many People Have OCD?" International OCD Foundation.
http://www.ocfoundation.org/prevalence.aspx

"How to Live With OCD and Use It to Your Advantage." Squidoo.com.
http://www.squidoo.com/how-to-live-with-ocd-and-use-it-to-your-advantage

"List of Foods High In Tryptophan." LiveStrong.com
http://www.livestrong.com/article/247974-list-of-foods-high-in-tryptophan/

"L-theanine for Obsessive-Compulsive Disorder." LiveStrong.com
http://www.livestrong.com/article/459424-l-theanine-for-obsessive-compulsive-disorder-ocd/

"L-tryptophan." University of Michigan Health Systems.
http://www.uofmhealth.org/health-library/hn-10006312#hn-10006312-uses

"Medicine for OCD." International OCD Foundation.
http://www.ocfoundation.org/medsummary.aspx

"Medicines for OCD in Children and Teens." International
OCD Foundation.
http://www.ocfoundation.org/meds_kids.aspx

"Obsessive-Compulsive Disorder." Anxiety BC.
http://www.anxietybc.com/parent/obsessive.php

"Obsessive Compulsive Disorder." KidsHealth.org
http://kidshealth.org/teen/your_mind/mental_health/ocd.ht
ml#

"Obsessive Compulsive Disorder." KidsHealth.org
http://kidshealth.org/parent/emotions/behavior/OCD.html

"Obsessive-Compulsive Disorder." National Alliance on
Mental Illness.
http://www.nami.org/Template.cfm?Section=By_Illness&Te
mplate=/TaggedPage/TaggedPageDisplay.cfm&TPLID=54&
ContentID=23035

"Obsessive-Compulsive Disorder." National Institute of
Mental Health.
http://www.nami.org/Template.cfm?Section=By_Illness&te
mplate=/ContentManagement/ContentDisplay.cfm&Conten
tID=7415

"Obsessive-Compulsive Disorder: Questions and Answers." The Child Study Center. http://www.aboutourkids.org/families/disorders_treatments/az_disorder_guide/obsessive_compulsive_disorder/questions_answers

"Obsessive-Compulsive Disorder: Tests and Diagnosis." Mayo Clinic. http://www.mayoclinic.org/diseases-conditions/ocd/basics/tests-diagnosis/con-20027827

"OCD and Severity." The OCD Centre. http://www.ocdcentre.com/sites/default/files/ocdseverity_1.pdf

"OCD: Rational People, Irrational Disorder." PsychCentral.com http://psychcentral.com/lib/ocd-rational-people-irrational-disorder/00012777

"Passionflower." University of Maryland Medical Center. https://umm.edu/health/medical/altmed/herb/passionflower

"Physical Activity Reduces Stress." Anxiety and Depression Association of America. http://www.adaa.org/understanding-anxiety/related-illnesses/other-related-conditions/stress/physical-activity-reduces-st

"Selective Serotonin Reuptake Inhibitors (SSRIs)." NHS.uk http://www.nhs.uk/conditions/SSRIs-(selective-serotonin-reuptake-inhibitors)/Pages/Introduction.aspx

"Self-Test." Beyond OCD. http://beyondocd.org/test
"St. John's Wort." Medline Plus. http://www.nlm.nih.gov/medlineplus/druginfo/natural/329.html

"Talking With Kids About OCD." International OCD Foundation. http://www.ocfoundation.org/ocdinkids/professionals/talking_with_kids_5-12yo.aspx

"The neuropharmacology of L-theanine(N-ethyl-L-glutamine): a possible neuroprotective and cognitive enhancing agent. " (2006). Nathan PJ, Lu K, Gray M and Oliver C. *Journal of Herbal Pharmacotherapy*, volume 6, issue 2, pages 21-30. http://www.ncbi.nlm.nih.gov/pubmed/17182482

"The Numbers Count: Mental Disorders in America." National Institute of Mental Health. http://www.nimh.nih.gov/health/publications/the-numbers-count-mental-disorders-in-america/index.shtml

"Treatments for OCD: Cognitive Behavior Therapy." Center for Addiction and Mental Health. http://www.camh.ca/en/hospital/health_information/a_z_mental_health_and_addiction_information/obsessive_compulsive_disorder/obsessive_compulsive_disorder_information_guide/Pages/ocd_treatments.aspx

"Treatments for OCD: Medication." Center for Addiction and Mental Health. http://www.camh.ca/en/hospital/health_information/a_z_mental_health_and_addiction_information/obsessive_compulsive_disorder/obsessive_compulsive_disorder_information_guide/Pages/ocd_medications.aspx

"Top Ten Jobs for People With OCD." Inside Jobs Blog. http://www.insidejobs.com/blog/top-ten-jobs-for-people-with-ocd

"Understanding Obsessive-Compulsive Disorder." OCD-UK.com http://www.ocduk.org/ocd

"What Causes OCD?" OCD-UK.
http://www.ocduk.org/what-causes-ocd

"What Is Not OCD!" OCD-UK.
http://www.ocduk.org/whats-not-OCD

"What is Obsessive-Compulsive Disorder?" Anxiety BC.
http://www.anxietybc.com/resources/ocd.php
"What is Serotonin?" Medical News Today.
http://www.medicalnewstoday.com/articles/232248.php

"What OCD Isn't." OCD Education Station.
http://www.ocdeducationstation.org/ocd-facts/what-ocd-isnt/

"What You Need to Know About Obsessive-Compulsive
Disorder." International OCD Foundation.
http://www.ocfoundation.org/uploadedfiles/whatyouneed_09.pdf

"6 Reasons Why CEOs and Investors Need Slightly OCD
Consultants and VPs." Workplace Confidence.
http://www.workplaceconfidence.com/tag/using-ocd-to-your-advantage/

"10 Things You Should Know About Compulsive Hoarding." PsychCentral.com http://psychcentral.com/lib/10-things-you-should-know-about-compulsive-hoarding/0006787

CPSIA information can be obtained at www.ICGtesting.com
Printed in the USA
LVOW01s2255170814

399621LV00016B/471/P